2020

2020

John Roman Baker

WILKINSON HOUSE

2020
Copyright © John Roman Baker 2020
The moral right of the author has been asserted.

First Edition June 2020
ISBN 978-1-899713-69-1

Wilkinson House Ltd.,
20-22 Wenlock Road,
London, N1 7GU
United Kingdom

www.wilkinsonhouse.com
info@wilkinsonhouse.com

Cover design: R. Evan
Cover art: artist unknown, Brighton ca. 1980

British Library Cataloguing-in-Publication Data
A catalogue record for this book is available
from the British Library.

All rights reserved. Without limiting the rights under copyright reserved above, no part of this publication may be reproduced, stored in or introduced into a retrieval system, or transmitted, in any form, or by any means (electronic, mechanical, photocopying, recording, or otherwise) without the prior written permission of both the copyright owner and the above publisher of this book.

CONTENTS

Part One
Knowing what is needed   7

Part Two
The past never leaves us   65

Part Three
Separate people   93

Part One
Knowing what is needed

The castle of his birthplace, the United Kingdom, had drawn up its drawbridge, sealed its doors, and like all enclosed spaces, it smelt, faintly to begin with, of the decay to come. He could not bear it. He would not bear it. It was to his only friend, Alan, that he expressed how he felt.

"I cannot live here any longer."

Alan looked at him across the café table in the North Laine where they had decided to pause after a long walk around Brighton.

"But this place inspires you. Look at what you have written."

"I disown it."

"Why?"

Alex stirred his cup of coffee, raised it to his lips and then lowered it again without drinking.

"Well?" Alan asked.

"I'm in my late fifties. I am no longer inspired. I just cannot be enclosed by cemetery walls."

"You can hardly call Brighton a cemetery."

"To me, it is." Alex paused, and then added, "Alan, you belong to this city. You have solid friends here. You are integrated, and you are younger than me. Perhaps in ten years or twenty, the city will be purer, cleaner, and the sordid will not display itself so openly on the streets as it does now. People will look again as they once did—with hope."

Alan cut into the cake beside his coffee with force and crumbs scattered over the café floor. He bent down and tidily picked up each crumb and placed them on a side plate. He looked at Alex and grinned: the boyish grin of a young man who had admired his work for years, or at least who said he had. Alex had lost belief in such easily said words.

"You are clean, at least," Alex said, responding to the grin. "You travel lightly, and you clean up on your way. Most people here are stuck down, glued to their mediocrity."

"Alex, please! You're in a bad mood. It will pass."

"Why should it?"

"It will."

"And anyway, why should I want it to pass?"

Alan pushed the cake aside, leant forward on his elbows, resting his good-looking head in the palms of his hands, and stared fixedly at Alex.

"Have you had another disappointing encounter on that dating site? Most of the profiles are phoney. You do know that."

"I have no illusions, Alan, and I only respond to people in other countries, the further the better."

"Well that's strange, what with you being a sexual racist, and not responding to people of other skin colours. A big mistake. I met a guy from South Africa recently, and he was very nice!"

Alex looked at Alan and played with the word *nice* in his mind. He had no experience of South Africa, but he knew that Alan was right. He did only respond to people of his own skin colour. It had been like that all his life, and he had taken it for granted that it was normal for him. He had no prejudices, no sense of racial hatred, he just knew what he liked, knew what he needed, and what he certainly did not need was the *nice* of this world. He had seen the *niceness* of England and now in a *nice* way it had turned particularly nasty. Racism, of course, was a part of it, but there were other factors as well. The elites of Eton and such places were in power and their *nice* smiles, used at times of crisis and terrible change, made him literally sick. *Nice* to him, was a person who had no knowledge of themselves, who lived on the basis of the persona of the self only, and who abused others who had any viewpoint that did not correspond to their own. They had sucked and become fat on privilege, and they charmed the vulnerable with all the *nice* etiquette they had learnt at their limited and violent schools. It was *nice* being passively violent to others; sacking people at whim. Alex knew that he was *not* nice, and that was why Brighton excluded him. The tight-arsed circles of culture and privilege had sniffed out too quickly that he was not one of them. He got more pleasure talking to the homeless on the streets than he did to those bathed in the still and rancid waters of English and American cultural theory. But Alan was talking, and he was not listening.

"Then there was my Columbian. He was so rich in his way of seeing and doing. I remember how before Christmas we went down and placed lighted candles on the pavement, and all his friends came from around the city. It was a magical party until the neighbours complained."

"Quite," Alex said. "You had disturbed their television with something real. And did he respect that?"

"The Columbian?"

"He had a name, surely."

"I can't remember. Javier, I think. No, maybe not. Anyway, let's call him Javier. He was polite, and we all sat in silence, no longer singing."

"So, you quietened down for *them*?"

"Javier was always polite."

"Poor Javier!"

"Alex, you are in a foul mood. Is it someone you have met? An Englishman by mistake? Instead of a Latvian?"

Alex smiled at the sarcasm. "It is no one but myself. My inner self says I have to force down the drawbridge and escape."

"We can never escape."

Alan got up to get more coffee. From the counter, he waved a plate of fluffy looking cakes at Alex. Alex responded by shaking his head in silence. When Alan returned to the table, he brought back on a tray, two coffees and a pink cake that epitomised the café they were in: stacked-up, highly-priced, pretentious confections that reflected the dead atmosphere of the surroundings.

"You know what your problem is?" Alan continued as he sliced into his second cake.

"Tell me."

"Romanticism."

Alex laughed.

"No, really it is," Alan continued. "You want what is elsewhere. Other. That is why no one much wants you here. You are an arrogant romantic. You make them feel provincial. And they don't like that. For a start, you go on too much about fucking Stendhal."

"What *is* that made of?" Alex asked, diverting the conversation.

"Slices of sponge, wedged with pink cream and fresh raspberries inside and on top." He said, his mouth full.

"And do you like it?"

"I suppose you think it's vulgar."

"No, Alan, just useless."

"How can you have a useless cake?" Alan asked, laughing, his mouth half-open, revealing pink mush inside.

"It just seems to me to sum up a lot," Alex said calmly.

Alan finished the cake quickly, then after delicately wiping his mouth, stared again at Alex.

"Look, my friend, this city is worth living in, and the work you have done writing about it is excellent, if a bit abrasive. Clearly, people in Kemp Town do not really live the same hedonistic lives you have described."

"No?"

"No. That's a bit of non-poetic license on your behalf. But never mind about that. It's sex you need. Meaningful sex. Not just a wank, staring at your computer screen."

"I don't."

"You don't what?"

"Stare at my computer screen. I don't wank anymore, full stop. My system has dried up. I look at a penis and think, yes for urination, yes for procreation, but not, especially not, for love." He noticed how shocked Alan looked at this observation.

"You've been reading too much French literature," Alan retorted.

"No, I have been reading *my* reality."

"Oh, I give up." Alan's grin had gone, and he pushed the remains of his raspberry cake away. "So, what is it that you need? You are like one of those dreadful riddles that can never be solved."

"Don't flatter me. I am not such a riddle. I simply want to leave a barren country for one that is connected to life. I want to see frontiers, not guarded by the sea, but frontiers of grass and roads. I want to know that I can travel from Calais to Vladivostok and never once have to cross that forbidding water. Water that drowns refugees. Water that drowns the hopes of the young who want to travel."

"Romanticism again," Alan sighed.

After a long pause, Alex asked, "Why do you bother with me? Why do you want to know me?"

"Because you are a singular person."

"Very singular. You haven't introduced me to even one of your friends. I feel like an intellectual older mistress living in some back street of your imagination." To his surprise, Alex saw Alan blush.

"You *are* older," Alan said quietly.

"Ah, at last! The truth! I have wanted to hear that for years. I don't smoke pot, I don't curl up on sofas and watch boxsets on Netflix, and above all, I do not go out on what is laughingly called *the scene*."

"Don't put me on the spot," Alan protested.

"But it's true, isn't it? That's why you don't introduce me to your friends."

No answer came. It was as if Alan was cradling himself in his polite shell. Inside that shell, he could not hurt others, or so he thought. Alex realised otherwise.

"I am giving up on friendship," Alex announced.

"What?"

The head popped out of the shell.

"You heard me."

"Even me?"

"Yes," Alex said with a sense of finality. "I don't want penises. I don't want that kind of love any more. Nor do I want platonic devotion that goes nowhere. Do you realise I do not even know your address?"

"Yes."

"Well, think about it!" Alex got up, placed a ten-pound note on the table and left the café. It was February and it was raining. Inside, he had left the city behind him. He wanted to be elsewhere. A stranger. He thought of Baudelaire's poem:

— *Qui aimes-tu le mieux, homme énigmatique, dis ? ton père, ta mère, ta sœur ou ton frère ?*

— *Je n'ai ni père, ni mère, ni sœur, ni frère.*

— *Tes amis ?*

— *Vous vous servez là d'une parole dont le sens m'est resté jusqu'à ce jour inconnu.*

— *Ta patrie ?*

— *J'ignore sous quelle latitude elle est située.*

— *La beauté ?*

— *Je l'aimerais volontiers, déesse et immortelle.*

— *L'or ?*

— *Je le hais comme vous haïssez Dieu.*

— *Eh ! qu'aimes-tu donc, extraordinaire étranger ?*

— *J'aime les nuages... les nuages qui passent... là-bas... là-bas... les merveilleux nuages !*

Yes, he wanted to see clouds. Passing clouds. Clouds high in the sky, low in the sky. Storm clouds and large cumuli that rise so high they make the earth itself look like something dead, lacking in supremacy. He needed the clouds of another country. There was no happiness to be found in the English cloud. The English would subjugate them all to their will if they could, and if the impossible were possible, demand passports from them and the right to stay.

Angry storms were battering England. Thick, sludge coloured clouds were wetting themselves over flat plains, drowning out houses, even in *nice* pleasant little places like Herefordshire where certain celebrities had their homes; celebrities mostly who could afford insurance and still happily raise the English flag against the storm. Agincourt had been won, even the failure of Dunkirk was a victory, so this storm could be won over as well. And then came the next, almost immediately. But England knew no defeat, because it was sovereign now, and like refugees in the sky, those dark invaders would be pushed away by American winds. All would be well, and the apple orchards would survive.

The storms provided the background to his decision making. He had to be totally honest with himself, and that was difficult, for like the variations of the wind and the rain, he too had variations. He knew that if he left the United Kingdom for another country, he would never return. Despite its failures and its self-destruction, he still had feelings for Brighton, having spent his childhood and much of his adult life there. Parts of the city had a resonance that he would miss and long to see again; the Clifton area he especially cared for. He had spent his late teenage years there. He'd had a lover in Clifton Road who was still alive but whom he had never seen again. With this man, he had learnt to love music, and thanks to him, he had met a woman artist who also inhabited this area of the city. She had died of cancer at the turn of the 21st Century, Even in the rain, while contemplating his possible departure, he walked those streets, recalling one memory after another, especially those evenings spent with his lover and the artist, listening to the latest music recordings and afterwards discussing their merits. Those had been tender years, and the white houses of those streets still held their beauty. As he strayed from this now very privileged area, he recalled the English master from his school, who invited him to his home in the furthest reaches of Hove and gave him books and encouraged him to write. Alex was an avid reader, absorbing superficially (how else does one absorb at the age of fifteen?) the complexities of life in Thomas Hardy's *Tess of the d'Urbervilles* and the flood in *The Mill on the Floss* which fed him the knowledge of narrative but not the interior lives of the characters. Why had brother and sister clung to each other in the flood that had drawn them down, clasped in an embrace? Why had Angel Clare been an object of desire for him in *Tess*, and why hadn't Tess's hanging for murder at the end of the book not left a more profound effect? A fifteen-year-old feels a lot but knows nothing.

"Write from the older person's perspective, not the younger. Try to understand how *he* feels," the English teacher had advised one day.

He had tried but failed. He *knew* how the younger person felt, but the other character who was twenty or so years older could not become a complex reality in his mind.

"I couldn't do it," he admitted. "Have I disappointed you?"

The English teacher who seemed very old to him but was probably only in his early fifties, smiled and said slowly, "You must learn to comprehend the world of others. You fail to describe him now, but you too will be that character's age."

"But I am not that age," Alex replied simply.

"I have just one criticism. Naturally, you cannot understand the interior lives of those who are much older than you, but you should have attempted to use your imagination, even though you would have probably got it wrong. You should have made a guess. However improbable your realisation on paper, it would have been interesting to read."

"Then shall I fail at being a writer?"

"No, not at all. But let's put it this way, if you do not grow in empathy; such deep empathy that all readers can go inside all the characters in your books, then on many levels your work will be second rate. The reader may well follow the narrative, but there will be a certain—how shall I put it?—disappointment."

The words had stung. The fifteen-year-old who was now in his late fifties, walked the streets near the long since dead teacher's house. How many people had lived in that house since? The area, near to Portslade, depressed him, and as he walked back beneath the darkened sky, he thought of another incident with the same man, when at the age of sixteen he had told him he was gay.

"Do you masturbate?" the teacher had asked.

The question came as a shock.

"Yes."

"And do you think of—?" The teacher turned his head away and looked at a bookshelf as Alex waited for the end of the sentence.

"Do I think of what?" he asked.

"Of boys? Men?"

"Boys, yes. Men, no." After saying the words, his instinct was to leave. "I'd like to go," he murmured.

"No, please don't. It must be a shock to be talking so explicitly with me. You look pale. I will make both of us some tea."

Alex sat reluctantly down, and stared at his locked fingers, locked so tightly that his knuckles were white. He also felt rather faint. By the side of the chair was a small table, and in his peripheral vision, he noticed the hand of the English teacher set down a cup and saucer. In the saucer were two biscuits. "Thank you," he said, but he did not look up, and neither did he unlock his hands.

"Drink it while it's hot. You look cold."

He unlocked his hands, and after a minute or two, still without looking upwards, he reached for the cup. He sipped at the pale liquid and then took one of the biscuits which he ate as quietly as he could. The room was silent and to him very cold.

"Now shall we talk?" the English teacher asked.

"I've said everything I have to say. I hope you are not judging me."

He heard laughter then: the laughter of a much younger man. The sound released Alex's emotions, and tears began to flow down his cheeks. With the back of his hand, he wiped them away. The laughter stopped.

"I remembered something," the teacher said.

Alex looked up and studied the man seated in front of him. He was smiling, and in his hands, he held a book.

"I am taking a risk here," he said slowly. "I would like you to read this book by Edward Carpenter. He is not read much these days. It's called *The Intermediate Sex*. It might help you. I know it helped me when I was your age."

"You mean—" Alex began but could not continue what he needed to ask.

"I had feelings like you, yes, but I trained them. It's a strange thing to say, but this instinct of ours for the same sex, can be tamed. Edward Carpenter lived in Brighton. He did not tame it, and he had a full and good relationship with another man. He had to leave Brighton. He needed a quieter life—a country life. He knew that Brighton corrupts. I too have retreated from corruption, but not from this town. I teach, and I consult myself; my inner self, and I have succeeded in taming my desire. I do not criticise Edward Carpenter for not taming his, but I respect his life for being a successful one."

He paused, and Alex saw tears in his eyes. Controlled tears. Alex noticed how blue his eyes were. They stared at each other for a long while in silence.

"Do *you* think it is a bad thing?" Alex asked.

"It is neither bad nor good. It is what you make of it. I try to see all things objectively."

"But God? The Bible?"

"God made us," the teacher said with a note of sadness in his voice.

"*Did* He make us? Does He even exist?"

"I think it is good to believe in God for as long as one is capable of believing." He got up, and going over to the bookcase, pretended (for Alex sensed that it was pretence) to look for another book. With his back to Alex, he said quietly, "I love Thomas Hardy most. I have read all his books, his poems. I find peace there despite the conflict of the characters—conflict sometimes resisted and sometimes not. You too will go through a lot of conflict over this matter of homosexuality, but in the end, you will know what is needed. Needed for you. Carpenter found what he needed. Many do not. I will be an old man one day, and I want to die with my conscience clear. I can accept the suffering of death, but not the mental pain. That, I believe, is the Hell that the Bible really describes. We are, you see, if we are not careful, our own instruments of torture."

"I don't quite understand," Alex said, and turning away from the bookshelf, the English teacher smiled.

"It's simple. So simple, many don't understand. Do not harm yourself and do not harm others."

"That's not so easy."

"No, it isn't. And that is why desire, the inflictor of so much pain, has to be tamed, has to be reined in like the charioteer and his horses."

"I am reading *Phaedrus* at school."

"It's a wise book."

Alex relaxed and leant back in the chair. He looked around the living room, perhaps really for the first time. There was no mess of paperwork or exercise books. It certainly did not look like a workplace for correcting school papers. "Do you have a study?" he asked simply.

"Yes. Upstairs. I will have to get on with some correcting soon."

This was a hint that Alex should go, and he stood up. "I am glad I told you," he said.

"Good. Can I suggest one more delicate thing?"

"Of course."

"I know at your age it is not easy, but try to resist masturbation as often as you can. Draw the energy up to your mind instead. Take down a book and read until the needs of your lower body pass."

Alex nodded his head, and as he did so, the teacher handed him the Edward Carpenter book, which had clearly been bought many years before and was almost falling apart.

"I want you to keep this. It's in poor shape, but it was much read when I was about your age. And do be careful who sees it."

Alex thanked him, and as he held the book in his hand, he felt in its touch the desperate touch of the persecuted all those who had suffered imprisonment for their desires. At school, a youth older than himself, whom he desired, had joked about the persecutions of the *fairies* as he called them. Alex had seen the hatred in his eyes as he recounted burnings at the stake, red hot pokers, and the declaration that any man like that should be put to death. He listened and he shuddered, but he still felt desire for him.

"You're looking very pale again. Are you taking care of yourself? There's a bad flu going around, you know."

The front door was opened, and Alex walked down the small pathway to the street. The English teacher waved goodbye to him, and the door closed. Alex put the book into his coat pocket. A few days later, he did come down with influenza, and when he recovered, he learnt at school that the English teacher too had been ill, and that he had died of pneumonia. Now, as Alex walked by the house, he wondered if he was guilty of giving the teacher the virus. He had tried to banish the thought for years, but it haunted him all the same. The English teacher. Why did he always think of him as being simply that? He knew his first name. He never used it with him, but he knew it. His name was Edward. He had known his surname as well, but now, years on, he could no longer recall it. There had been so many other names since he had been that teenager: so many surnames and Christian names written down in lost address books or on scraps of paper. He should have been remembered Edward, but one thing Alex had learnt was that memory only returns to us what it chooses, and that is certainly not always what we want. Edward, and Edward Carpenter. He had read most of Carpenter, and when he did, there was always a man behind the books: a sort of ghost or shadow which cast its light and its darkness over the pages. Initially, he had found Carpenter's writing strangely dull, considering that it had been given to him to help him understand his homosexuality. The language was not his, but a few years later he found one of his lesser-known books: *The Art of Creation*. He had it still, and even if he left everything else behind, he would take that book with him. There is a reason for loving certain books that only the inner self knows. How many books he had read in his life, absorbed, and then later been unable to recall their content? He even forgot the content of some of his own books.

"Daydreaming?"

He was deep in thought, sitting in the over-crowded café of St Ann's Well Gardens. When he looked up, he saw Alan gazing down at him, smiling. "Would you like to sit down and have a coffee with me?" he asked.

Alan looked wryly at him and murmured, "Still friends?"

"Familiar acquaintances," Alex replied, and then got up and ordered two cups of coffee. He thought of buying Alan a cake, but there were only rock cakes left, and he saw them as a symbol of the English heart. He waited for what seemed an age for the drinks to be made. When they came, he returned to the table and found Alan with a copy of The Guardian open in front of him. "Can you find me one article about men in it?" he asked as he placed the coffee in front of Alan.

"Don't be cynical. It is only right that they should spotlight women's issues and champion them more than the other rags."

"Yes, but—"

"No, Alex. Stop this phoney anti-this, anti-that. I know it's all said for effect. Can you wonder that I am the only person in Brighton who is fond of you?"

Alex sat down, facing him. "Fond? Rather a strong word, especially from you. It's a neighbour of love, fondness. No. You are not fond of me, Alan. You like my mind. You like to squeeze it like a sponge." He paused, and then added, "I still think you're a bastard not to have ever invited me to your house or introduced me to your friends, even though they're all so young. There are so many gay places we could meet up in, or would it be too much of a risk to your image to be seen with me?"

Alan closed The Guardian, folded it and put it into his pocket. "I am sorry," he said.

"No, oh no, please do *not* be sorry. For your own reasons, I am to be kept to one side. If you were sorry, you would change that."

"Alex, shut up."

Alex did shut up and waited for Alan to bring the conversation back to life.

"The truth is, and this you won't like, Alex, I like older men's company, especially when they have a mind like yours, but I don't want people to get the idea that they are lovers of mine."

"So, you don't want to meet me socially because they might think you suck my cock?"

"Please, Alex!"

"No, please yourself. Oh, let it go. It's all coming to an end anyway."

"So, you are—?"

"If you mean leaving the country, yes I am. I have just enough money to buy a simple house in France."

A group of children began to play Cowboys and Indians noisily around the table, and Alan looked dismayed. The gunfire and Indian war cries continued for quite a while until a woman, immersed in a mobile phone conversation, called them back to their table. As she continued her conversation, the children took up their game again in another corner of the café.

"Are you shocked, Alan, that kids still play games like that?"

Alan blushed. His blond features were very prone to blushes. "It's so—"

"Morning television, Alan. Something you may not know about, but they still show Westerns on obscure channels. All retro, preceded by politically correct warnings. I saw one a week ago. The Indians fell like flies." He paused. "Now what shall we say to each other?"

"Have you really made up your mind?"

"Yes, Alan. For the last time, yes. And my choice is France. You know I love the country, and there are small towns and large villages with houses going for £55,000 or even less. I couldn't buy a corner of a sewer in this city for that price."

"But how would you survive in a place like that?"

"I speak French fluently. I read French. I'd get by. I'll have just enough to live on until I get my pension which, as long as Boris Johnson wasn't lying, has all been agreed. But who can be sure? I will be 59 in a few months. I can hold out."

"On what you earn from your books?"

"That will help. Fortunately, the Australians, the Americans, and even the French read me. You may, deep down, think I write trash, and that I have only written one good book, years ago, but you see, those moronic, empty-headed homos who read me, lap it up. They are not so concerned about Roland Barthes or being philosophically correct."

"I don't only like one of your books. I like your poetry."

"Fuck my poetry."

There was silence between them. The children came back to play, and one of them pointed an invisible gun at Alex. "Bang!" the little boy cried out.

23

"Well, there's an honest little boy," responded Alex, patting the top of the child's head. The child screamed and ran back to his mother, crying, "He touched me. That nasty old man touched me."

Alex looked towards the mother and smiled, mouthing the words, "Sweet child." The mother nodded her head and then returned to her phone.

"Have you decided on a particular town or village?"

"Only the area."

"Can I know?"

"I'm afraid not. Not yet. You have too many things on your mind to remember a French provincial name, and I'd look rather a fool if it all fell through."

"You've seen some places on the web?"

Alex nodded and said he was on the brink of going down to investigate.

"Send me a postcard, if you do," Alan said, and without another word, he got up from the table and left Alex to himself. The rain had begun again, and Alex watched as Alan walked over the rather muddy, sodden grass and was soon out of view. St Ann's Well Gardens had never seemed quite as depressing as now. Alex felt a tug on his sleeve.

"Has your friend left you alone?"

It was the little boy who had shot him earlier, accompanied by an even smaller child.

"Yes," Alex replied.

"Did we make too much noise?"

"No."

"My brother and me, we like games. We play all the time. Did you used to play once upon a time?"

Alex smiled down at him and said that yes, he had played a lot with life.

"How can you play with life?" the boy asked. He had black hair and big questioning dark eyes.

"It's an easy game. You will play it one day. But then night comes, and it is all over."

"Silly game," the boy said, not unkindly.

"Very silly," the younger boy behind him echoed.

Alex looked down at them, and for a moment he was shot through with fear. A voice inside him was screaming with pain, and the silent words cried out, it's too late, it's too late, it's too late.

The day Alex decided to travel to France, the trains to London were messed up, and at Gatwick Airport he had to get off and was told he would have to wait.

"How long?" he asked the conductor.

"Someone on the line."

A woman jumped forward, between him and the conductor and said spitefully, "I expect it's a suicide. This line is made for suicides. They love to drag us all into their own deaths."

"Madam, I can assure you it is not a suicide."

"That's what *you* say," she said, and moved back into the small crowd.

The rain was pelting down, and Alex felt quite hopeless and lost. If this was an omen for a new life, it was not a good one. Who knew what the person was doing on the line! Then as he stood on the crowded platform, he had a sudden, irrational dread of the Coronavirus that had already seen a few cases in Europe, and a feeling of panic gripped him by the throat. Images of men he had seen die in the past flashed across his mind: men, isolated in their beds, dying, and no one knowing what was happening, or what was going to happen. He cried out and separated himself from the crowd. A young man who was nearby, came up and touched him on the arm.

"You alright?" he asked.

"No," Alex replied. "I am afraid. I was going to find a new life, and now I am sure I will never get there."

"Far away?"

"Yes."

"Not a good time to travel. I mean, this virus—"

"I'd better go back to Brighton. Maybe I should get a taxi."

"No need for that. I am waiting for a Brighton train. We can travel together."

"Yes," said Alex bleakly. He looked at the lines of rain as they fell, perfectly straight, relentless. "Will this never stop?" he asked.

The young man laughed and looked at the rain as well. "Never rains but it pours."

Alex smiled at the cliché, and the stranger took his arm again.

"You look terrible. Sit down. Here, I have a flask with me. You need a hot drink, and don't worry, I haven't used the cup!" He poured out a cup of hot coffee and gave it to Alex who drank it down in short but frequent gulps.

"You're kind," he eventually said. "I'm Alex."

"I'm Paul. Nice to meet you."

There was an awkward silence and the rain, blown by a change in the wind, started to fall at an angle, hitting them.

"Let's find the right platform," Paul suggested. "I'll carry your suitcases for you. Is it just these two?"

Once in the train, Paul stared at Alex as if he knew him, and Alex was momentarily embarrassed. What does he see in me? He wondered.

"Said you was going on a long journey, didn't you? What with all this hold up I may have got things mixed up."

"I was going to Paris," Alex said quickly.

"Not that far then. Not like India or Japan. Easy to get another train on another day." Paul replied and looked out of the window.

Hesitantly, and with a note of absurdity in his words, Alex asked what Paul thought of the state of England.

Paul laughed and stretched back in his seat.

"Bloody fucking awful. I come from the North. Live in one room in Brighton. It's bloody hard." He paused. "But I voted the bastards in. Can you believe it? Me, a socialist and I voted them in. All because I didn't think the other lot were up to much. I must have been drunk in that polling station."

"Where did you vote?"

"Don't ask. I'm too ashamed. God knows why I put that cross in the place I did. They said to me, it will keep out Farage. I did it for that." He paused. "Did you do the same?"

"No. Green. No other option where I live."

"I've only been in Brighton for a month. I was on my way to Clapham Junction. Training for a new job. Then this."

"Maybe you will be able to bear it. This country."

"What do you mean?" Paul asked.

"I think you will live with it."

"Do you think I'm simple or something?" Paul's voice sounded cross, and Alex realised yet again that he was not fit to be among people. He was terrible with his jibes and in his tone. He aroused anger in so many.

"I should mind my own business," Alex said.

"S'alright. I ain't angry, but people think I am stupid. I read books. I know things. Just can't make friends."

Alex smiled at him and asked spontaneously, "Will I do? Will I do as a friend, even if it is temporary?"

Paul glanced down at his hands. The train lurched, and looking out of the window, he said, "I think we are going too fast." Then, turning to Alex, he replied, "Never had a male friend. As for women, I'm not interested. Never have been. Can't trust 'em."

He likes to talk, Alex thought. I should have sensed he was— He stopped on the word: the word that made categories and built walls. This man Paul was perhaps reaching out to him, but he had so little time. You have a goal, he reminded himself. He felt like a rusty key which no longer knew how to turn a lock, open a door.

"Come to my place for a drink?" he offered.

"Thanks, I will," Paul replied.

A silence of relief separated them. Unbelievably, the key had worked.

They could have taken a taxi on arrival at Brighton, but

instead they walked in the rain. On arrival at Alex's flat, Paul surprised Alex by asking if he could take a shower. There was no hint of sexuality in either Paul's question or his tone of voice, so Alex showed him the bathroom and made some drinks and snacks. As he did so, he heard the sound of the shower and of water splashing in the bath. He pictured the large yellow bathmat getting soaking wet and figured he would have to put it over the radiator to dry out afterwards. After a few minutes, the noise stopped and Alex, sitting on the sofa with two glasses of whisky and a couple of sandwiches in front of him, waited.

"That's better," Paul said as he came into the room, looking at the food and drinks on the table, but not at Alex. "I needed that. It was cheeky of me to ask, so thanks."

Alex handed him the whisky.

"Will warm me up. I had a cold shower and a cold bath. Always do. I hate hot baths."

"Why?"

"As a kid, my mother always forced me into very hot water. No escape from the heat or the steam. A steamy room with no ventilation. I've hated it ever since."

Instead of sitting beside Alex on the sofa, Paul sat on a wicker chair as far away from Alex as possible. Alex found Paul's behaviour strange. Either he wanted something, or he wanted nothing. Usually, he could make out the signals, but this time he could not. The atmosphere between them was not at all the same as it had been in the train. There he had sensed the beginnings of a confession, but now he sensed the impulse had gone. Paul sipped at his whisky cautiously and in silence. He had not touched the food. Eventually, the silence between them became oppressive.

"Do you like music?" Alex asked.

"Do you?"

"I asked first."

"It's not really necessary for me. I'm passed pop music, and I get disturbed by—the bombardment of classical."

"I thought it would have been the other way around."

"Maybe."

Silence again. And then, like a bolt from the blue, Paul asked, "Are you lonely?"

Alex had no idea what to say. Officially he was; he had no friends, and there was only one acquaintance left: the discord between Alan and himself. He tried to define quickly within himself what loneliness actually meant. Was it a relief to be unwanted after all? Was it a clean space not to have anyone think they had a right? And yet—

"I was told long ago to control the need for others," he replied. "I had to train myself."

"Who told you that?"

"A lover. He died. Alone. He showed how much control he had. The nurses said that even with the minimum of energy that he had left in him at the end, he fought them all off."

"Sad story."

"Is it?"

"Yes."

With a gesture near to impatience, Alex pointed to the table.

"Please eat a sandwich. It's only chicken and salad—all I had left. You must be hungry."

Paul went to the table, picked up a plate and took just half a chicken sandwich. He seemed to be acting out of politeness and without desire. He was being obedient to Alex's request, and there was a certain insolence in the way he moved. I will do it because I have been asked to do it, but I am no slave to any order, Alex thought. Then he returned to the wicker chair.

"So, what are you planning to do with your life?" Paul asked as he bit off a corner of the bread.

"This country is making me ill. I want a new start."

"Won't France make you ill as well?"

"It's a risk."

"At least you know what you're up against here."

Alex watched as Paul put the hardly touched food down

beside his chair. He had also hardly touched his drink. Did he imagine Alex had spiked it while he was out of the room? As if to reinforce these thoughts, Paul asked if there was any beer instead.

"I thought whisky would warm you up."

"Beer is what I feel like. Out of the bottle. More like home."

"I didn't put anything in the whisky, if that is what you are thinking."

"How would *you* know what I am thinking? I'm used to beer straight from the bottle!"

Alex was not afraid of this hostility. God knows he was used to it. "Throw the glass at the wall if it makes you feel any better," he said.

"All I asked for was a beer, and now you think I'm thinking things I wasn't. I suppose you're going to ask me to leave."

"No."

"Why?"

"Why? Why? Why? Why anything? All people do is ask why, including you. Why do I want to live in another country? Why don't you ask why I am breathing?"

Paul laughed at this. "The air is the same in Europe. Do you believe you'll have more reason to live if you breathe it there instead of here?"

"Yes, I do."

Paul seemed to get quite excited, as if he were enjoying this sudden burst of interrogation, of argument. Alex wondered yet again why people always wanted this from him: this hostility that would eventually alienate them. Was there nothing in him that implied the possibility of endurance, of mutual lasting and wanting? It was not that he had a low opinion of himself, only that he had something within him that repelled rather than attracted. Few people had been indifferent to him.

"So, to return to my leaving. I have been rude. Isn't that

enough for you to want me to go?" Paul asked.

"You seem different to how you were on the train. You even talk different. What accent is that?"

Alex stood up, and Paul took over his place on the sofa. He lounged back against the cushions, his legs wide apart, his penis clearly delineated beneath the cloth of his trousers. Alex had not taken any notice before. It did not excite him, but it fascinated him. Clearly, Alex thought, Paul had omitted to put on his underwear after the shower. So where was his underwear now? In the bathroom? He resisted the urge to go and look.

"I was tired on the train. Tired of the rain. I'd stood in it longer than you. I still feel damp. When I'm tired, my accent comes back. Hull. Makes me sound ignorant down south. Useless. The lad who knows nothing and will never know anything. Been to Hull?"

"No."

"It's cut off. Lethargic. No proper trains. Successive governments have cut us off more and more from the rest of England. Almost an island. I guess like you, I don't like islands."

"Islands can be beautiful," Alex said, and went to pour himself another whisky. "But this country is not my kind of island anymore, just as Hull is not yours."

"So, we do at last have something in common."

"I forgot your beer," Alex said, retreating to the kitchen. As he reached for the bottle, he thought, I am old, or fast getting there. He's young, but I don't feel even a twinge of desire. He can't be any more than thirty. He could well be younger. His hair is dark, not thinning. His body is slim, almost too thin, and his face is lined and drawn as if he has been on a fast for months. Sharp lines cut down from his eyes to his mouth, and his chin is weak and a little puffy, and yet he is an attractive man. He has the eyes of a wolf. I like wolves. His eyes sparkle with mischief and life, and there is just the hint of ginger in them; a hint that the ferocity of the redhead is somewhere within him. These thoughts were cut short as Paul appeared beside him.

"Got a nice flat here," Paul said as Alex handed him the cold bottle.

"My whole life is crammed into this rented space. My books overflow on the floor. The pictures have accumulated over the decades. The rest is in storage. It's the colour that makes the place look good. Without that, it would be a white shell and quite dull."

"You like the arts?"

Alex felt in no mood to talk about paintings, books or anything related to culture.

"I like certain works that people call art, but art, in itself, is a fraud. I do not collect, I just keep what I like, not what I ought to have."

Paul put down his beer and applauded. Long, slow applause.

"We have a good art gallery in Hull. The Ferens. I used to go there. Just sit in a room, choose a painting and stare. The best place in Hull is that gallery."

Alex sat at the kitchen table, and said, "I'm glad you responded like that, but please can we not talk about art. I want to get away from it—all the useless artefacts men gather around them: the picture that is only there to be the envy of those who come to dinner. All that fraudulent nonsense kept out of vanity, never necessity."

"You talk like a writer."

"I am a writer."

"So, you collect words."

"No, I use what I know. I don't pillage dictionaries to convince critics or acquaintances to give me good or at least not bad reviews. There is no honesty in publishing anymore."

"I wouldn't know." Paul sat opposite Alex at the table, and his question was very simple, "What is it you reject, Alex?"

Alex stared at the long, glinting eyes. He could tell that the question was sincere.

"Three things fail in life. Three. They are what we consider the essentials. Do you know what they are?"

Paul shook his head.

"Society. It always fails. Love, and I include friendship in that—that too fails. And the third is aesthetics, or so-called art in all its forms. The third is the worst, because it pretends to give you visions and a state of otherness, but once absorbed like a strong drink, it dissipates in the system. For example, I like to listen to certain operas. What heights and depths they pretend to take you to—and then the plunge. They leave you lonelier than ever before because in all art is the pretence that society is real, that you can work with it, live in it, but that destructive thing called society, does not permit that. It even forces the dead to pay for their non-existence in what false society call funerals. As for love and friendship? Art encourages you to want it, like a whore who shares so much, promises so much, but in the end, withdraws. And what do human emotions really relate to? You're there to prop up another's ego, or if you are the needy one, you need a faithful person to tell you how you are, how you are within, when there is no access to anyone's heart or soul."

"You're in hell," Paul said.

"We're all in it," Alex replied.

"Not me. That's for sure. I get myself around this society, and if it's going to get worse, it's just a bad storm to ride, like what is happening out there with the weather. As for love, well, I've had affairs, good ones as well. I have no complaints. And art? I just read a book I like and don't get too involved. I know it's fiction, and that's that. As for paintings, I get high on colour."

Alex smiled at Paul and then asked if he wanted to go or whether he'd like to stay for a meal with him. Paul said he would like to stay, and after the meal, and watching a film on television, Paul revealed more about his life.

"I lied earlier. I wasn't going up to London for training. It was an interview. Well, the train screwed that up. It wasn't for anything spectacular. Shop work. But better than what I'm doing now—part-time in cafés. It's bloody hard living in Brighton. I've got a room in a house bulging with people—out Moulsecoomb way. Not a place to take you to. I live on a pittance. If I'd got that job, I'd have had to have moved up to London, but that's fucked now."

"I'm sorry," Alex said.

"Life's shit, but unlike your theories, there's no pattern to it. Shit is just a messy splurge, and so is life. But you can get out of the muck if you try. I am still trying. I don't think you should give up on England and move away."

Alex was silent. He heard the words, but Paul's truth was not his truth, and he wanted quite simply to find himself alone in a place where a border could be crossed, and another language could be spoken in freedom. He wanted to escape the prospect that on the 31st December, tight controls would weigh down upon the UK and so many things he had taken for granted would be taken away from him. Taken away by people like Farage, Johnson and Cummings who were now so much in control.

"You can sleep on the sofa, Paul. I have extra bedding. We can talk some more, that is if you are not working in the morning, and if you like we could go somewhere tomorrow, just for the pleasure of it."

"On what money?"

"Don't worry about that. We may never be real friends, but I don't mind helping for a while."

Paul smiled. Then his smile turned into a wide grin, and his eyes shone as if some long-lost father had given him an unexpected present.

"No strings?" he asked.

"Definitely not, but I have to ask." Alex grinned also. "What happened to your underwear? It's obvious you are not wearing any."

Paul looked down at his groin, and then still grinning, stared at Alex. "I just didn't want to put them back on after my shower. They smelt. I put them in the washing basket. Sorry."

"Don't worry. I've got some spare clothes. I just want you to feel comfortable. Now, I'll get the bedding."

"Don't *you* have to work tomorrow?"

"My last book was still-born. I don't want to create another."

"You need inspiration."

"No, Paul, no. Just a new life."

The bed on the sofa was made up, and Alex was about to leave the room when Paul came up to him and kissed him on the cheek. It was a light kiss, but Alex felt uncomfortable with it. He did not need the human touch of mouth or hands.

"Sleep well, Paul."

He closed the door to the living room and made his way to the bedroom. Can I trust him? He asked himself. Supposing I wake up and find something gone? He smiled to himself as he got into bed. Less for me to take, he thought.

The following day, Alex took Paul to Rye. It was the only place he wanted to revisit, perhaps for the last time. As the train pulled out of Lewes, the small talk they had engaged in after leaving Brighton stopped. Alex looked at the Downs, so magnificent as they gently sloped into the distance, and he thought of Paul. He still had so much life ahead of him. From zero to fifteen, we are children, and from fifteen to thirty, we are young men. Then from thirty to forty, we are in our prime, and following that from forty to sixty, we are middle-aged. Finally, from sixty to eighty, we are old men. That is the mathematics of it: the inexorable mathematics of life. He was travelling with a man still in his youth, while he, Alex, was on the doorstep of old age. As he stared, he thought of the Downs, living their seasons, and he knew, finally and hopefully once and for all, that he wanted to walk by soft rivers, to live on a plain in France, and to die near trees. As a young man, he had caressed the folds of the Downs like a lover, but now he was tired of climbing the heights to see distant valleys or witness the life of villages below as one does on Devil's Dyke. Climbing up and tumbling down, making love in the clefts of grass and chalk. He had felt that youth was forever, because from the age of fifteen to thirty you believe that youth is forever. Now he needed the flat plains and their eternity. He needed the tributaries of the Loire and to see, until his eyes finally darkened, the simple church towers, and to hear the tolling of distant bells. Old age is the flat prelude to life's ending, and to him the plains symbolised that in their quiet relation to earth and sky.

"What are you thinking?" Paul asked.

"The obvious. That you are young and that I am approaching old age. It's strange, but it is true for me that the Downs always remind me of the journey to come. One downland invites another, and like the legs of youth, the journey appears to never end. The Downs do not understand this because of course finally they fade into the sea. I have walked all I shall on the Downs and am ready for the simple plain that has no undulations but whispers that you can remain on one spot: the comfort of knowing there is nothing to seek out or to claim."

Paul stared at him and then turned his head to look out of the window.

"That's all very poetic," he said, "but I don't really understand all of it."

Alex smiled at this.

"You can smile," Paul persisted, "but all this nonsense of old age and resting in one's spot! Do you really mean what you say, or did you get it from some book? I believe that until we die, there are always more places to see, other things to confront, and high places to climb. There are obstacles at any age. You can't honestly believe that standing on a plain is not going to bore you. I thought you were more realistic."

Alex opened a guidebook and handed it to Paul. "What's

realistic?" he asked. "Perhaps you'd like to read up about Rye."

"And no more nonsense talk, okay? I came out with you for a break."

"I'm sorry. I don't want to spoil your fun."

Paul flipped the pages over, looking at the pictures, then handed the book back to Alex.

"I'll see it when I come to it." He paused and then asked, "Why is this place so special to you?"

"Because it's a part of my visual past that I will be leaving behind. For example, from the tower of the church, you can see the beginnings of Romney Marsh: a place like no other. Some people call it one of the wonders of the world."

"Why?" Paul put his head in his hands, his elbows on the table and stared at Alex. Outside, the sun was shining—a brief day of respite from the storms and the rain. Alex saw the ginger in his eyes glitter as if caught by a ray from the sun. He looked eager.

"I can't answer your why. You'll have to go there to find out if it is true for you."

"Then let's do it, Alex. Let's go to Romney Marsh."

"First Rye."

"But doesn't the train go there?"

Alex paused, and then said, "Yes, alright, we will try to visit Romney Marsh, but first Rye. We can spend the night there, and if the weather holds, we can catch a train to Appledore tomorrow."

"Is that the next stop down the line?"

"Yes. From there you can get to Fairfield and an ancient church in the marsh called St Thomas à Becket. For me, it holds the very essence of the marsh."

Paul leant back in his seat and grinned. Then he said he had to go to the toilet, and after a while, he returned, and stood looking down at Alex.

"Train's almost empty. D'you think people are getting afraid of travelling? Or maybe no one wants Hastings or wherever." He then stretched himself and yawned. "About this church. I'm not much into religion."

"You have to see it in its context. It stands alone with a wide expanse around it. It has a magic. If you look again at the guidebook, there is a picture. You can see what I mean."

"Well, if that's the essence of Romney Marsh, I think I'd rather we just spent the day in Rye."

"Why have you changed your mind?"

"Oh, spending the night. I can't afford it, and I don't want you to pay for it."

"But I paid for the fare. You didn't mind that."

"I know, but that's the limit, plus maybe a drink and a sandwich in Rye, but I don't want you spending more money on me."

"Not even if it gives me pleasure to show someone the one place in this country that I truly love?"

Alex sat down. The glitter had gone from his eyes, and he looked sullen.

"Someone? I have a name. I know we are strangers. We haven't even known each other for twenty-four hours, but I hate to be referred to as *someone*—as if I am the last person in the world for you to clutch onto."

"That's unkind," Alex said softly.

"No, it's not. I can't fill a temporary gap before you go back to your solitude. I thought about it in the toilet. You are using me, Alex."

Alex was at a loss to reply to this, and then said, "You're right. I am using you as another pair of eyes to see a place I love. The only place I will miss. Isn't that worth a night? With separate rooms."

"It will cost a fortune," Paul mumbled.

"I can manage it."

"Lucky you!" There was a sneer in Paul's voice as he said this.

Alex went through his pockets and brought out four fifty-pound notes. He placed them in front of Paul.

"Let me give this to you. As a thank you present. You see, Paul, I am perhaps pretending, but I thought I had met a new friend."

Paul reached out and touched the notes.

"I'd feel like a whore if I took them. I can't. It would be one of two things. It would either be a debt, or payment for spending a couple of days with you."

"A whore would ask for a lot more than a couple of hundred."

Paul shouted at Alex. "I'm not taking it. I'd feel dirty. Don't you understand I'm ashamed of not having money?"

The train stopped at a station. Neither of them looked out to see where it was. Paul glanced at Alex, and then started panting as if fighting for breath. His face was white with anger. No one got on the train, and it moved off again.

"Why don't you just hit me and get it out of your system?" Alex asked. "I can see you want relief. You look ill."

"You're right. I am. I get panic attacks, and you're about to tip me into one."

"I certainly don't want that," Alex responded lamely.

"Oh, sod your fucking Romney Marsh!" Paul cried out. "And I lied. I do like old churches." He got up, and stumbling away from his seat, muttered, "I'm gonna pass out, I know it. It's all spinning."

Alex got up, but Paul had already run down the aisle of the carriage and locked the toilet door. There were retching sounds from within. Alex knocked on the door. There was no answer, and now he began to panic. Supposing Paul had passed out? You could die on your own vomit. He fought back the terrifying thought and sat down facing the toilet door. The train stopped at Hastings. A few people got on but went into the next carriage. It seemed that providence was giving them their privacy. He was tempted to seek help, to unlock or kick in the door. There was a guard on the platform, but it was too late to call out. The train started up again, and Alex looked out at the sights of the town: houses built upwards on the cliffside in what seemed for a fraction of a second to be a foreign town. Then the toilet door clicked open. Unsteadily, Paul came out, and before Alex could say a word, he said, "I'll take the money. I want to see the church."

Alex turned away from him and walked slowly back to the place where they had been sitting. Paul followed him, and they sat in silence for a while.

"You gave me a scare," Alex said, looking now with indifference at the scenery outside.

"I should accept," and reaching across the table that separated them, Paul touched Alex's arm.

"What should you accept?" Alex responded, turning to face him.

"Your offer. Your kindness."

"I'm not kind."

"My head cleared in that stinking toilet, and I could see how this whole country stinks at the moment. I know too that the stink won't go away. The bastard landlords that are allowed to rob us, and the minimum wage pay-by-the-hour employers; they depend on us to still tip our hats to them, just like it was before we got some kinds of rights. And Brighton is rotten with all that, despite what our MPs say, and the speeches they make in Parliament. We are slaves. Suddenly I understood why you want to get away from this slavery." He paused here, and his voice sounded choked. Alex looked into his eyes and saw tears. Tears that did not fall but were there.

"Then you do understand why I need to get away?"

"Yes, but haven't they got problems like we've got here? Supposing all is going well for you in whatever town or city you choose, and that woman gets elected? I can never remember her fucking name."

"Marine Le Pen? You surprise me."

"There you go again, assuming I'm simple because of my accent. I can be a fool though. I don't know why I voted the way I did. Most people in Hull stuck with labour. I feel so bloody guilty about it. For example, in the street where I used to live, right next door there was a Polish couple. They had a kid, ten-year-old, and some of the other kids in the street used to spit at him, call him names, and say things like how he would grow up and steal their jobs. They daubed shit on their front door. Animal shit. And the little cunts wrote in it, 'Get Out.' Of course, they left. They had to leave. No, I don't understand much about politics, but all the stupid newspapers, and all the news on television had pushed them to hate the so-called *other*, and they pushed me to vote conservative to 'get Brexit done' and to keep the Farage lot out."

Alex looked down at the table. The train had slowed, and he felt totally empty. He had nothing to say, not really. He disliked Brighton in different ways, but not like that. Eventually he said softly, "Paul, this country has always hated the *other*. Napoleon should have invaded and left us with some decent laws."

Paul laughed at this. "You don't mean that," he said.

"No, I don't. Invasion and war are terrible. But the English have this fear of being ground down by the *other*. These past few years they have felt invaded by Europe. They want their freedom, their independence, and they cannot see the new invisible chains, and how they will be invaded again—not by Poles or Romanians, but by others and—" He fell silent.

"I know," Paul said.

"Stay and help fight the wrongs. That's what you probably think I should do. Or don't you?"

"You can't run away. You can walk away, but you can't run away."

Alex smiled at this, and reaching into his pocket, he silently handed the money over to Paul. Paul took it, looking at the notes for a while as if he might change his mind again and refuse them, but eventually he put them into his trouser pocket.

"I suppose we'll be there soon," Paul said.

"Not far."

"At least the sun is still shining."

"We will only have a few hours of daylight there," Alex observed.

"You going to take me up that church tower?"

"St Mary's church. Yes. The view is—"

"—spectacular. I know. It would have to be for you to love it."

Alex was puzzled by the way Paul's mind worked, and how he could appear indifferent one minute and enthusiastic the next.

"You sound very positive about it suddenly."

"It's the only place or person you still love here, isn't it?"

"You make me sound very poor, aside from money."

"That's none of my business," Paul said, the words coming out coldly, and despite their intimacy on the train, Alex knew they were still strangers.

They arrived in Rye on time, and as they left the train and made their way out of the station, Paul commented, "The air smells—well, sweeter than Brighton, not stale. I bet you have to be bloody rich to live here."

Alex smiled and said nothing, and for the next hour, he showed Paul significant houses, and talked about the people who had lived in them: Henry James, Rumer Godden, and E.F. Benson. He mentioned that apart from Godden, they all had same-sex feelings. Paul passed no comment, but when they arrived at the Catholic Church of St Anthony of Padua, he refused to go in.

"Let's not," he said. "It's such an ugly building."

Alex then told Paul about Radclyffe Hall and how she had paid for a cross in the church and dedicated it to her former lover Mabel Veronica Batten. He was talking about *The Well of Loneliness*, when a priest came out.

"Won't you come in?" he asked, smiling.

"We're short on time," Alex replied. "I was just telling my friend about Radcliffe Hall."

The priest gave them both a withering glance and Paul, noticing it, said very loudly, "She was a famous lesbian. I believe she donated the large cross inside and that it is dedicated to one of her lovers."

Without another word, the priest turned and hurried down a path next to the church.

Alex did not know whether he felt embarrassed or not, but he respected Paul's cry of defiance.

"Was I too strong in calling her a lesbian?"

Alex smiled and said, "I'm ashamed of myself, Paul. I could never have used the word lesbian out loud like that."

"Well, according to you she was. I believed you. Wasn't she after all?"

"No, she very much was!"

"And the book they banned. Was there lesbian sex in it?"

"Only a hint at it, but that was enough to create a scandal at the time. People used to smuggle it in from France. The ban lasted for many years."

"We're a prejudiced lot, aren't we? Is it better to be gay in France?"

"In some ways, yes, in others no."

"That's no answer, and please don't walk so fast. We don't have to escape from that church just because of what I said, do we?"

"I want us to see the view from the tower."

"You're not answering my question. Is it better there? Do they have gay marriage?"

"Yes, they do, but there was a great deal of resistance and more public outrage than here, but deep down the French accept what you are. They are a complicated race, but you have the right to privacy and to be who you are without interference. Unlike this country, homosexuals were not imprisoned. Oscar Wilde spent the last years of his life in Paris, after he was released."

"I didn't even know he was released. That's good."

"Yes and no. He died in poverty."

They were walking slower now, and Paul said quietly, "I don't want that to happen to you. I'm afraid for you, Alex. I mean, your age is not exactly on your side, is it?"

"Thanks for the reminder that I'm an old man."

"Well, you are, but you're young too."

Nothing more was said.

On arrival at St Mary's, they entered by the north transept door, and Alex paid for them to go up the tower. The way up was arduous for Alex with all its twists and turns, and the risk of falling. He clung on to Paul more than once and was panting when they stepped out into the light at the top. It felt cold, and Alex huddled into his coat. Looking sideways, he saw a look of surprise, almost joy on Paul's face.

"Wow. I've never seen anything like it." He pointed with his finger. "Is that Romney Marsh?"

"Yes. Marred a little by the—"

"—don't say it. Those wind turbines give us energy for the future." Reprimanded, Alex started to point out some of the buildings below, but it was the distant view that appealed to Paul: the marsh and its landscape, the winding waters of the Rother glittering in the February sunlight. "It's all silver like the scales of a fish," Paul commented. "And the marsh, it looks like a place that goes on forever, like a fairy tale."

"There is a poet in you, Paul," Alex said.

"It's what I see. It's as simple as that. Aren't I right?"

"Now you know why I love this view and the marsh." As Alex said the words, he recalled the feelings he'd had the first time he had visited the tower years before in the eighties. It had given him comfort and a sense of splendour that this place and the magic that emanated from the distant marsh was able to dispel his fear of Aids. He did not mention this to Paul. He kept these thoughts to himself, and yet, despite the beauty of it all, he felt cold.

"You need a cup of tea," Paul said, turning to Alex, his lean, marked face glowing as if it had been burnt by the sun. Passion, Alex thought, can do that, pushed outwards from within, released from an unidentifiable place of imprisonment and given freedom to the body and soul. He longed to feel what Paul clearly felt; the newness of life that comes from an overwhelmingly good experience. He glanced down once more at the scene below him, but like Paul, his eyes were drawn beyond the buildings towards the river and the marsh beyond.

"I'll come back here," Paul said as they began their descent.

Once in the street, they made their way to a nearby teahouse, and while they waited for their toasted sandwiches and tea, Paul investigated the contents of a bookshelf that was filled with books people had apparently left behind.

"They're being sold off cheap. For charity," he called out to Alex. "Good titles too. I remember reading the Hornblower books when I was a kid. I guess I must have a bit of the sea in me."

"Did you ever see the film with Gregory Peck? They shot that here in Rye."

"Did they?" Paul exclaimed. "Anyway, they've got a combined edition of three of the Hornblower books on the shelf."

"Buy them! You'll enjoy rereading them."

"I haven't got any change."

"Then use one of the fifties I gave you."

"I meant of my own money."

"But I gave that money to you."

"Yeah, but it's your money, not mine. I would like to buy out of my own money or not at all."

"Paul, the money I gave you *is* yours."

"Did I *earn* it?" Paul replied with a snarl in his voice.

"This is a fuss about nothing. I've got some pound coins in my pocket."

Paul stood up and said, "I don't want them, and I don't want this." He then took the money Alex had given him out of his pocket and returned it.

Their food arrived, but neither of them ate what was put in front of them.

"That money was a gift, Paul," Alex mumbled, and the cold he had felt on the tower returned inside him. He knew now that Paul would want to return to Brighton and that they would not visit the church in the marsh. "I suppose you want to go back."

"I couldn't stay here now."

"Paul, I was only offering some small change."

It was a last throw of the dice, but the dice, as usual, did not fall in a positive way.

"Please shut up about it, Alex. You've given me a great day out. I loved the view. I will never forget it, and I owe you for that, but now I feel it would be better if, instead of separate rooms, we went our separate ways."

"I thought by now we were sort of friends." The words came out with difficulty, and the three things that fail in life (for everybody?) flashed across Alex's mind: society, love and friendship, and finally, art. Even the view of the marsh from the tower was now tainted in his mind.

"We know a lot about each other, Alex, and I appreciate your kindness, but we are not in a relationship."

"I said, in the train, I am *not* kind!"

Paul got up and said, "Shall we go?"

With a sense of hopelessness, Alex got up, went to the till and paid for the meal. He found Paul waiting by the door. Suddenly, he no longer cared. He was leaving the country. He would shut himself away in a place of his own, a place that would have all its doors closed.

On the way to the station, Paul tried to make casual conversation, but Alex had nothing to say. He was in the shell he had made for himself.

There was a long wait for the train, and while Paul hid himself in a waiting room, Alex walked up and down to keep himself warm until, without warning, he felt tears fall down his face. There had been a sudden break inside of him, and he covered his face with his hands.

On the train, Paul produced his own small guidebook to Rye. He said he had found it in the waiting room, and after lingering over a few images of the town, he murmured, "There are so many places we missed."

"Yes," Alex replied flatly. He felt that Paul was trying to provoke him somehow, but why?

"I'll have to come to Rye again," Paul said quietly.

Alex leant back in his seat and looked at Paul's face. He looked tense and pale, and Alex wondered if he was close to another panic attack. He knew he had to respond and that he had to try to stay calm until they reached Brighton.

"So, what did we miss, Paul?"

"The Mermaid Inn. That's where they filmed the Hornblower film you were talking about."

"Was it?" Alex replied. "I didn't know that."

Paul reacted to this by saying, with rising anger in his voice, "Of course you knew. Why lie to me? I don't like being lied to. You know everything about Rye. You told me so."

"Stop it, Paul," Alex cried out. Too bad if he has another vomiting session in the toilet, he thought. I won't worry. But of course, he knew that he would.

Paul raised his hands up, and for a brief second Alex feared he would attack him, but instead Paul tore at his own hair. Then as suddenly as he had begun, he released the grip of his fingers and lowered his hands to his sides. "I feel ill," he said.

They were quiet for a while.

Alex glanced out of the window. It was now totally dark outside, and he saw his own reflection in the glass: a worried elderly man. He turned away from the image of himself and almost whispering, said to Paul, "Mermaid Street is the most beautiful street in the town. That's what most people say anyway. Personally, I like the small streets around St Mary's church. There is a certain peace there, which I find special."

"Yes," Paul replied. "I like them as well." Then he asked, "Would you really have taken me to that street and the

Mermaid Inn?"

Suddenly, a strange thing happened within Alex. He felt emotional pain. Paul had got to him. His voice had sounded like that of a child. He felt as if he wanted to sit beside him and comfort him as a sincere friend comforts another.

"I was going to take you after we'd had our tea."

"Really?"

Alex could read the question in Paul's eyes quite clearly. They were asking, are you telling the truth?

Excusing himself, Alex said he had to go to the toilet, and he made his way into the next carriage. The two women who were the sole occupants were talking loudly, and he heard one of them asking the other, "Do you think this thing from China is going to take hold here?" He did not linger to hear the reply. Stress was building in him, and he did not want to contemplate a possible panic or the world turning into chaos. He wanted a retreat so he wouldn't have to see the hell that Brighton could become. He knew only too well that the government wouldn't care how many people died as long as they could protect their own interests. Reaching the next carriage, he flopped into a seat and thought, I must not show pain. I must not be drawn into emotional feeling. I will refuse all pain once I am gone from here; once I have taken that one-way journey out of this wretched country. I lived in Paris for many years. I was young. I was happy. I won't find that happiness again, but I do need contentment: the peace you feel when the savage pulse of life does not beat so fast. He closed his eyes. He had to reflect on those six years he had spent in Paris and why he had returned to his so-called home, which had given him nothing but disillusionment. Even as a child, I sensed the roots were rotten, he thought.

"Alex." Paul was standing over him, looking concerned. "Why did you run away from me?"

He hovered over Alex, and Alex felt suffocated by the shadow of his presence. He did not reply at first and thought, I must never, ever be in this kind of situation again. I have finished with the ways of men: with their charm and attraction, with their hatred and their ferocity. I only want business transactions, like dealing with estate agents and signing papers. No more of this tension, of never knowing what the other feels.

"Can I sit with you?"

Alex nodded his head.

"Another empty carriage," Paul said. "Did you hear those women talking about their fears?" Paul was still standing, and Alex could not bear the shadow.

"Please, for God's sake, sit down," he said.

Paul made a movement to sit next to him but paused and instead chose to sit opposite. It was as if he sensed no touch was welcome.

"I heard them," Alex said.

"Are you afraid?"

"I have a sketched portrait in my flat, made by a young artist many years ago. It's a man's face. At least, I assume it to be a man, but the lower half of the face—the mouth—is not there. At the time, I thought it romantic; just a sweep of hair flowing sideways, as if underwater, and the deep impress of the dark eyes. I found the lack of the lower half of the face mysterious, but now, since the last few weeks, all I can see is a doctor wearing a mask."

"Are you going to get rid of it?"

"I don't know. It's beside my bed. I am not sure what to do with it. It seems to be waiting."

"Don't say that. The virus will be contained. It's not a pandemic."

"Can we not talk about this, Paul?"

Paul nodded his head and looked outside. The train was drawing into Hastings. "Never been here either," he said casually.

"I got off once to stretch my legs. In the distance I saw the castle on the hill. 1066 and all that."

"Yes, the Normans. Didn't need passports then. At school

in Hull, they said it was the only invasion this country had ever had. What a load of bollocks. We've always needed fresh people and for different races to mix."

At Hastings, they had to change trains, but Alex was tired. When the train for Brighton arrived, they found their seats and Alex closed his eyes and tried to block out the sounds of the other people getting on—the high-pitched voices and the rough voices he always associated with the unkind. He drifted off to sleep, and the sleep was a black void. He awoke when Paul told him they had arrived in Brighton.

"Already?" he said, and he wiped his dry eyes. A few people around them were gathering their things together, but Alex did not want to move until they had gone. "Let's wait until the passage is clear," and glancing at Paul he again felt a stab of inner pain. This is not going to end here, a voice said inside him. He shook his head as if to deny the thought.

"I've something for you," Paul said.

Alex watched as a piece of paper with a row of numbers was handed to him. He took it in silence, knowing what it was.

"Mobile number," Paul said.

"Yes," Alex replied, and then he did what he thought he would not do. He took a scrap of paper out of his own pocket and wrote down his own number. The one thing he had no desire to do, and yet had to, and he did not know why. Paul took it without comment.

They got off the train and walked in silence to the exit where the pungent smell of urine hit them. Paul noticed it first and said, laughing, "Welcome to Brighton." Alex gave him a wry smile.

"We'll say goodbye here," Alex said.

"Thanks for the day." Paul held out his hand.

So far, there had been no more than a minimum of physical contact between them. Alex noticed how firm Paul's grip was. The grasp was held a little longer than necessary, and while Alex felt the heat of Paul's fingers, he heard him say, "I'm sorry. I always fuck things up. I just didn't—"

Their hands unlocked, and Alex replied, "No need to say any more. We saw the view from the tower."

"Something to remember," Paul said, and then, without saying goodbye, he walked away. Alex stood and watched as he crossed the road and disappeared into the distance.

Alex could not go back to his flat. He carried on walking down to the Clock Tower and then turned left into North Street. The night was cold but clear. Tired as he was, Alex continued walking until he reached St James's Street. He gave some money to a young homeless woman who was huddled in a doorway. She had no teeth and grinned at him with an empty mouth. The look in her eyes was one of utter hopelessness. She mumbled some words, then bunched up her fists and covered her eyes. The gesture was so fierce, she looked as if she wanted to extinguish her sight once and for all. He walked on. A group of drunks were singing loudly, their clothes too thin for the cold. He continued his ascent up the street, and there, coming towards him was Alan. Alex opened his mouth, intending to greet him, but as he approached, Alan lowered his head and passed by without acknowledgement. He knew he had been seen. It was clearly a snub. The young man, who so liked Alex's mind, had finished with him.

Further up the street, Alex entered the Bulldog pub. A few scattered men stood like statues of flesh and stone. No one moved. Their eyes were as extinguished as those of the homeless woman. He approached the bar and ordered a beer. When it came, he downed it quickly.

"I'll have the same again," Alex said.

Silently he was given the beer, and one of the statues came to life and stood next to him. He pressed his body against Alex, and Alex edged himself away quickly.

"Excuse me!" the man said. He too looked tired, and he

looked old. He has lived for centuries, Alex thought. Centuries of endurance and probably solitude. But all the same, he wants to let me know that he is real, that his flesh bleeds and hurts.

"Don't apologise," Alex said.

"What's your name?"

"Alex."

"Alexander?"

"Yes, but I prefer Alex."

"I'm Ned. First time here?"

Alex did not want to lie, but he did anyway. "Yes. I came in just for a drink. I'm travelling."

"Travelling?" Ned laughed. "It's not a good time for travelling. February is the month to be still. Just get through it."

"A philosopher," Alex remarked.

"Am I? I don't think so. Just a bloody fool to be out here instead of at home. I only live a few streets away. As you are travelling, why don't you come and travel over to my place? I haven't eaten. Have you?"

"No."

"Then I'll make spaghetti. It's been, well, I don't want to bore you with my life story. Why are we born to become stories of ourselves? That's a philosophical question. See, I've got a brain," and he tapped his head.

"I have to go back to a friend," Alex lied again.

"Lucky! Does he make good spaghetti?"

"Sometimes, when he makes the effort."

"So, tell me, if you think I've got a philosophical brain, why is it we all create stories about ourselves? Lies, truths, all this inside of us? This jumble sale of events and things that happen to us, suffocating us inside? I suppose it all ends with death. Do you think it ends with death? That the stories disappear? All the ridiculous and sometimes good things, gone?" He snapped his fingers.

"I have to go," Alex said. He felt as if his head would

burst. Why did I come in here, he thought. I don't want the touch, the talk of men, and yet it seems I am drawing myself back into that human pool. I will drown. But I have to be nice, to him, to this man Ned, and smile at him, and go.

"Ned, next time I travel this way, and you are here, we will have that spaghetti."

Ned waved his hands in the air dismissively. "No, we won't," he said. "You won't be back. Travel. Travel. It's the curse of this new century."

"Yes, Ned, it is." Alex reached out and touched him on the arm. "Now, I really must go."

"Yes," Ned said and turned away from him.

Alex walked slowly out of the Bulldog, gulping in air, but it made him feel dizzy. The day had been too long, with too much high emotion. He longed to leave England and find peace: a peaceful solitude away from the disturbances that men inflict. Why had he not gone back to his flat, and instead gone to an area where he would see other men? The dilemma of contradiction is strong within the self, and however much reason says, yes, you can endure, you can be among others and separate from them, there was still as this night had proved, an urge, he could not fully explain, to embrace the presence of men like himself. And the most perverse thought of all, as he wandered back down St James's Street, was that he had actually regretted not sharing spaghetti with this lonely and much older man. He had not asked his age (how could he have?) but the whole stance of the man was that of a man in his late seventies, and yet, he was alone among the figures of flesh and stone to become truly flesh with the flesh's need to reach out towards another. Ned had chosen him. By the time he reached the Old Steine, he knew he had to go back to the pub. He had to say yes, and not no. He knew a person like Alan had many years ahead of him before the sands of time would run out, but Ned? He was astonished that he was thinking of another in this way. Ned was seated by a window when he re-entered the Bulldog, and without hesitation, Alex went up to him.

"Is that invitation still good?" he asked.

Ned looked at him warily. "Sit down," he said.

Alex sat at the table, and once seated, he looked closely at Ned's face. He saw that he was silently crying.

"What's wrong?" Alex asked.

"Since you left, I've been thinking about my life. I've had many lovers—how impossible I was to live with! I was so vain back in the early sixties. I was good-looking, and I changed lovers like others changed clothes. I had unsafe sex throughout the seventies and well into the eighties, and still I escaped becoming a casualty of Aids. I've no idea why. Then came the guilt of the survivor. I've seen my body deteriorate, and once last year I had a bad influenza that nearly finished me off, but I pulled through. I have a degree. I read a lot. I was once a good businessman, but now it's all gone." He laughed and then started coughing. "Don't worry, it's not the killer virus—just a leftover cough from an ordinary cold."

Alex listened to the litany of the man's existence. He was sharing the bones of his life, and how he had been reduced to those bones, and he was blaming no one but himself.

"I can still laugh," Ned said. "I laughed all the way through *Judy*. Do you think she was anything like that?"

"I haven't seen it," Alex replied. For once in a long while, he was not going to show his contempt for camp. Camp made others richer in their lives, but for him, it detracted. He would rather sit down and watch a Godard film than a flamboyant musical or a gay comedy. Not that there was much that could be called comic about Judy Garland's life. He knew that much. The difference in their ages meant that Ned had had her as a part of the fabric of his gay life, and he, Alex, had not.

"She sang all the songs herself—that actress. I liked the one from *I Could Go On Singing* the best, and I wept buckets when she sang *Over the Rainbow* at the end. In my imagination, I was right back there with that audience. Everyone there must have known she was at death's door."

"Can we talk more about this over spaghetti?"

"You said you were travelling."

"I lied."

"To get away from me?"

"No, Ned. To get away from human contact. I am, how shall I say, conflicted."

"Bisexual?"

"No, certainly not that."

"Well, you come back to my flat. I am glad you changed your mind. We will be there in a jiffy, and I will make you the best spaghetti you have ever eaten."

Ned wiped away the remains of his tears, and uneasily got to his feet.

"Cramp," he said. "I get a lot of cramp. I live in Devonshire Place. Ground floor, thank God. It's my own. No rent to pay. I may not have made successful lovers, but I made fairly successful money."

"What did you do exactly?"

"That's hush-hush. You would probably despise me if you knew."

The uphill walk to Devonshire Place was clearly a strain for Ned. He paused and panted several times and tapped at his chest often.

"Too old to go out on a cold night like this. And sure as my imminent demise, it will pour with rain tomorrow."

Finally, they arrived at Ned's flat—a 1950s Regency Brighton nightmare.

"Admit it. You stole everything from the Royal Pavilion."

"Except the kitchen! I have a brand-new kitchen." He paused and said, "You probably hate all this once-upon-a-time-long-ago Brighton tat, but it means something to me. I imagine I am back in time. As a promiscuous teenager I got seduced in so many houses and flats like this, and they nearly always played *Lucia* or *Norma,* when I wanted Cliff Richard. Oh well."

Alex thought Ned looked much younger in his home.

There was colour in his cheeks, and beneath the trademarks of old age, he saw the young man who was so proud of his looks. He envied him for having a place that had this effect of rejuvenation.

"Can I put on one of your CDs?" Alex asked.

"Take your pick."

"Have you any French singers?"

"Let me think. Yes, I've got Edith Piaf, Jacques Brel and Francoise Hardy. I can't understand a word, but I like the sound. Brel is too melancholic, so how about Francoise Hardy? She's a favourite. Do you know much French?"

"Yes, I know the language."

"Are they sad songs?"

"No, not especially. They're about how love can be happy and how it can change everything, for good or bad."

"Well, I never knew," Ned sighed.

Alex was about to comment on Romanticism when he saw, mixed in with Ned's collection of popular singers, a recording of Mozart's last two symphonies."

"Can I change my mind?" he asked.

"Just don't choose the Brel, please."

"Mozart? The last two symphonies. Can we have those on?"

Ned looked at him and then at the CD. "Isn't it a bit heavy for dinner?"

"Even if it's on quietly?"

"You listen to it while I prepare food in the kitchen. But first some wine. Only plonk, I'm afraid. Australian. Well, it can't always be French, can it?"

Ned went briefly into the kitchen and after a few minutes returned with two glasses of white wine on a tray which he placed on a side table. He looked at the CD player as if the music offended him.

"You might be interested in my collection of books. I hate having anyone watching me cook, or helping me which is even worse!"

Alex took his glass of wine and sat on a sort of chaise longue: a reproduction from a very uncertain period. Ned went back into the kitchen, and after Alex had listened to the 40th Symphony, and the 41st had just begun, he went to look at Ned's bookshelf. It was full of novels he had never heard of, mainly from the late sixties and early seventies, but further down a shelf of gay books caught his eye: Gordon Merrick's *The Lord won't Mind* and an American edition of *Dancer from the Dance*. He had read the Holleran, but the book had meant nothing to him as he had felt no identification with the characters or the decadent and purple-tinged prose that they inhabited. He returned both books to the shelf, and his glance moved to *Giovanni's Room*. This was a book he had admired years ago, but he wondered whether it could have any meaning now. Most of the titles seemed to have come from America. He noted authors like Jay Little and James Barr. As with Andrew Holleran, he presumed these were pseudonyms and had a feeling that Ned would know if he asked. Finally he spotted Gore Vidal's *The City and the Pillar*, in fact, two copies of it: the first edition from America and the revised one, a paperback, but among the whole collection there seemed to be no European writers: no Genet, no Alberto Arbasino or Hervé Guibert. These were the authors that had most influenced him. Arbasino's *L'Anonimo Lombardo*, published in English as *The Lost Boy* was his only work to have been translated, and Alex regretted that his other books had not been accessible to him. But then he noticed the exception: Carlo Coccioli's *Fabrizio Lupo*, translated as *The Eye and the Heart*. For a few years in Paris, he had read it and re-read it until his Livre de Poche paperback had almost fallen apart. But after—and here he had to shut out the thought of *after*—as emotion began to hit him in waves of self-disgust and horror. He could not and absolutely refused to think of what he had done. He balanced himself precariously against the bookshelf, and it was in this state that Ned found him.

"You alright?" he asked.

"I was just looking at your books."

"Well, it looks as if they have brought you to the point of collapse. Personally, I must admit, I don't read much now. I seem to lose concentration. I'll be seventy-nine next month, and they all seem a bit remote to me. Did you find my special books on the lower shelf?"

"You have quite a collection," Alex said, his breathing shallow. He saw again that face, the very young face of—and he pushed the name back—the force of doing so almost made him faint.

"I think you need some of my spaghetti desperately," Ned exclaimed. "I'll prepare the table, and you go back to the comfortable place you were sitting. Prop yourself up against the cushions."

"Wine before a meal always does this," Alex said, but in his mind, there was still the faintest image of that face and the lingering of the word *after*.

"You should have told me not to give you wine," Ned said.

Alex returned to the chaise longue. The Symphony was coming to an end. Ned busied himself putting out side-plates, glasses and mats, and in silence, he glanced over to Alex as if making sure he had not passed out. Alex, with eyes half-closed, wondered if Ned was afraid he might vomit over the chaise longue. The CD came to an end, and Ned gave an audible sigh of relief.

"Shall we listen to Celine Dion now?"

Alex no longer cared who they listened to, and making conversation, he asked Ned if he had enjoyed *Titanic*.

"Who could have resisted Leonardo DiCaprio back then? I hoped it would be Kate Winslet who went down, not him. Everyone in Brighton was in awe of the that young man, so sadly puffy and deteriorated now!"

"Are you sure I can't help?" Alex asked, suddenly desperate to do something, and above all, to end the meaningless conversation they were drifting towards.

"Relax! Food will be on the table in a jiffy. It's not my best spaghetti as promised. Certain ingredients are missing, and the wine isn't quite the right wine, is it? But then, this is all wonderfully impromptu, and I feel I am not alone. It's a good feeling to be making a meal for someone again, and with such a handsome man." He paused, fork poised. "I just hope we can become temporary friends. It would make me happy."

Ned returned to the kitchen, and Alex watched him, initially feeling sorrow for him and then refuting that feeling, sensing he that he had had a long life and that there was nothing to feel sorrow or pity about. The very old should never be pitied.

The meal was eaten slowly, and conversation wavered from one subject to another. Alex reflected on the day spent in Rye. What was Paul doing now, he wondered. Ned jolted him back into the present moment by asking a direct question.

"You are handsome but getting on in years. Are you alright, financially? I mean, Brighton is not a cheap place to live. Do you have property?"

Alex realised it was time for truth.

"I am semi-retired."

"So soon? How?" and Ned put down the fork that had held the last strands of spaghetti.

"I have a regular income, Ned. Enough to live here, but with no extravagances. I rent a flat and live off an inheritance my mother left me when she died. It was more than I had expected, and if I'm careful, it will last me until I get a pension."

"That's lucky—but then again, how unfortunate you could not buy a place. It so eases the mind, you know."

"I know," Alex replied, staring at Ned's concerned face. "I taught English in various foreign schools for many years. Then I needed to return here, to the city of my childhood and early youth. Unfortunately, this Brighton is not the Brighton I knew then."

"Yes, we've been battered by so many economic gales. That's why a shelter of one's own is so necessary."

"I know," Alex said simply and drank some wine.

"That's the second time you have said, *I know*. But what *do* you know?"

"I see a city heading towards destruction: the division between the rich and the poor widening, and a cityscape that in far too many places looks as if it is rotting away. Marine Parade, the mess that is the Western Road, the horror of the Lewes Road with yet more ugly places for students, and underneath, a cynicism that Brighton is somehow moving forward, and yes, for certain people I imagine it is."

Ned smiled. "What a speech," he said. "I suppose you read the Guardian and blame it all on the Tories."

"Labour is to blame as well," Alex replied, "but please let's get off politics. We may argue, and I've had a terrible day already. I am, Ned, what is called a social disaster—at least by Brighton standards."

"Oh, pooh!" Ned exclaimed, and standing up, began to clear the table.

"I must help," Alex said, feeling claustrophobia settling in.

"Certainly not. A guest is a guest. And you may not want to believe it, Alex, but I like you, and please, please do not worry that I found you attractive in the bar. I have passed beyond that rather tedious illusion and now see you as a man worth knowing. You have principles. We may disagree on politics, but I too see the shoddy state of this once glorious city. I have a simple question that it seems nobody can answer. Maybe you can." Ned put down the plates he was about to carry into the kitchen and sat down again.

"What is it?" Alex asked.

"Why is it that when I was a child, during that dreadful post-war period, this city looked so much better than it does now? The West Pier and the Palace Pier were both operating. The seafront was alive with flower gardens and coloured lights all the way along. Some things, of course, needed a bit of paint, but all in all, it looked great. I used to sit with my father and mother on seats facing the sea that were not rotten.

The Royal Pavilion too was a blaze of colour and light, as was the fountain in the Old Steine. There was pride despite the poverty. Maybe it is just a fantasy of my childhood years, but the town glowed, and its centre held. Brighton was Brighton, Hove was Hove, and both towns competed and were perfectly kept up." He stopped for a moment and then added, "And now that we are a wealthy country, the city looks shoddy, and the place has lost its heart."

"I wasn't there, Ned," Alex replied, "but I can believe it."

"Plus all the wonderful cinemas: the Astoria, the Savoy, the Odeon in West Street, not to mention the Regent and the Essoldo. And what have they been replaced by? Television and the internet."

Alex felt a genuine warmth coming from Ned. Even though they might never be able to become friends, this had been a good encounter; like a chance meeting on a ship. Once the ship reaches land, you make promises for it to continue, but it rarely does. He liked Ned. He felt he could open up to him.

"Ned, quite simply, the place has been slowly fucked up. And not many people are left to recall what you saw. They passively accept the *now* of the place. As for the rich, well, their gated fronts cut them off from the realities that you and I see."

Ned got up, brushed a sentimental tear from his eye, and took the dinner things back to the kitchen. Alex did not interfere. He knew Ned wanted to treat him as a guest, and he respected that. When Ned returned, Alex asked him if it was time for him to leave.

"No, please stay for a while longer. I have a selection of liqueurs. Fancy one?"

Alex nodded his head, and Ned opened a cupboard door to reveal an extensive selection of alcohol. He reeled off a list of names like a rollcall and asked Alex what he wanted. Alex laughed and said, "Whatever you have will be fine with me." He ended up with a delicious raspberry liqueur from France.

"So, you can really live off your inheritance without problems?" Ned asked.

"It's not easy, but I am careful. I've even put enough aside to hopefully buy a small house in France, in a village perhaps. I'd like to find somewhere in the Sologne region. One of my favourite books is *Le Grand Meaulnes*. It was *his* favourite book."

"His? Who is he?"

The drink, which was refilled, was loosening Alex's tongue. How quiet the flat was. He felt trust. Ned was not an Alan, or like some of the others he had had so-called friendship ties with. He was that rarity. A good man.

"He was long ago," Alex murmured. "A pure boy who made the mistake of meeting me. Luc. I don't want to go into details now, but this book of Alain Fournier's was our lovers' Bible. Often after making love, we would read chapters from it to each other."

Ned's eyes opened wide, as wide as a child's.

"Did he come from this place you mentioned? How did you call it? *Sirloin?* Is my attempt at French acceptable?"

Alex smiled, "Perfect."

"Don't flatter. But did he come from there?"

"Yes. Close to a place called Vierzon, which is in the very heart of France. The area is full of marshes, small lakes and tall, magnificent trees."

"And you love this place very much?"

"Yes."

"What a beautiful story."

Ned was a little drunk by now, and his eyes were slightly glazed.

"Forgive me if I don't tell you all of it," Alex replied.

"Alright, but tell me about this book with the impossible name. Can I buy it?"

"I'll pop a copy of it through the door. There's an English translation called *The Lost Estate*. The original title *Le Grand Meaulnes* is impossible to translate. It has too many layers.

Meaulnes is a young man, a teenager, who falls in love with a girl he sees when he gets lost one day in the countryside. I won't tell you more because it will spoil it for you."

"It sounds like something out of Hans Christian Andersen."

"The first part of the book is utterly magical. A dream. A fairy story. All that is best for the child in us, or the young lover in us."

"Were you *that* much in love with him?"

"Yes," Alex said. Then getting up, he went over to the bookshelf. The drink, the warmth, the slight headiness he felt was stabbing at his inner self. And just to recall Luc was like a hammer blow inside of him. He knew he would never see him again, but with luck, he could live in his country.

"You look so sad, Alex. You know, if you are ever hard up, you can ask me."

"Ned, Ned," Alex whispered, and then he went over to him and placed a hand on his shoulder. "I couldn't take from you even if I needed the money."

"But why?"

"I'm fierce on independence. I have to stand alone. Really stand alone, and yet, I like you so much because you are a giver and not a taker." He released his hand, and Ned smiled.

"I think I am too tired to go to bed. I think I will sleep on the chaise longue. I'll make up a story about your love for this boy. I'd love to write a romantic book, but I can't express myself on paper. Romantic books are wonderful. Look at all those titles on my shelves which the snobs would call trash. Yes. I will invent my own story from what you have told me."

"Make it better than it was."

"That's a strange thing to say."

"I mean it. Make it bright. Make it a blaze of light like you saw as a child when you looked at the Pavilion and the fountain in the Old Steine."

"Yes," Ned said. His eyes closed, and Alex realised it was now time to go. "You won't forget to bring me the book,"

Ned mumbled.

"I'll put it through the door tomorrow. What is your second name?"

"What's in a surname? Everyone knows me as Ned. Just put that on the envelope, or better still, ring the bell. You'll see Ned written under it."

"I'll say goodnight and show myself out."

"No, you're a guest."

"Stay where you are and then move to the chaise longue. Dream for me."

Bending down, Alex kissed Ned on his forehead.

"Like you," Ned said, eyes closed.

"Like you too. And thank you for the evening."

Alex recalled Paul thanking him at the station for the day spent in Rye. Despite their failures, despite the panic attacks and the hurts inflicted, he had thanked Alex. He kissed Ned's forehead again, and after putting on his coat, he made his way out of the flat.

Outside, the rain had returned. Alex hurried back down St James's Street and found a waiting taxi. He looked across at the unlit fountain on the Old Steine and the now austere garden that surrounded it.

"They're letting this town go to ruin," he said.

The Taxi driver turned and asked him what he had said.

"Nothing. I was thinking of the past," Alex replied.

Part Two
The past never leaves us

Alex knew that the past can only be remembered in fragments. It cannot be recalled at will. There is no way that he could question his self and ask, what was I doing in October 1983. He knew where he was, but he had absolutely no remembrance of any particular day. Yes, I went to Paris, he thought, and then came a silence of the mind as if a soft blanket had covered all memory. Luc. He had said his name to Ned. The love of his life? Who would he name or call for during the last moments of his life? Would Luc's face be the final image he would see before the void engulfed him? He thought it would more likely be something insignificant like tying up his laces for the first time as a child. But memory brings unwanted gifts, and those laces on his shoes might well be the final image of his life. He asked the ridiculous questions that all philosophers have asked since thought became active: how do we get to the strange place of all that has happened to us, and how do we sift through and bring out the gold and not the dross? The place was inside. All philosophers knew that, but the location of retrieval and the determining of whom we thought we loved most is locked within, and the key not available to open the way to recall. He could say, Luc was the love of my life, but what did that really mean? The day they met for the first time, what words were spoken? He should, if Luc was this tremendous love, be able to remember that conversation, but all he saw was two people walking hand in hand along the lower level of a *quai* in Paris, the name of which was lost to him. Perhaps there was a bridge and the looming bulk of Notre-Dame ahead of them. No, there was only the splashing of the River Seine as a *bateau mouche* passed by, and a bright light suddenly, bright enough for him to look closely and to stare at Luc's face. Fiction. It was all fiction. There had been in all probability no bright light and no bateau mouche, and no darkened edifice of Notre-Dame, only a quai on the lower banks of the Seine, and that they had held hands, of this he was sure. It was not a creation produced by his mind. The hands were definitely joined. The look had been given even if there had been no light to illuminate them. He cried out to himself, "Luc is gone," and the wail inside of him seemed to come from an invisible box of memory that refused to reveal its contents. No, I must go back further. I must unravel what comes to mind, and yes, like a novel, I will create the rest that does not reach the surface. I will use and force the consciousness of what I *can* remember and clothe it with false memory. I will fabricate, and that might do it; it might do what all the philosophers have failed to do, to open up the hidden domain where all lost souvenirs of time can be brought out. I must plunder myself like a pirate. After all, aren't all the words said, and all the actions made, inscribed within and written down? For the words to make sense, it is simply a matter of connecting them to intense sensations of pain and joy.

He had first arrived in France in 1979. The month was August. He could not recall whether it had been hot on the day of his arrival or a day of unusual cold. He had seen many days in many Augusts when leaves could be scuffed, and the sound crackled in his heart because, for him, it was a joyful sound and not one of sorrow. The first golden leaves. Impending autumn. In his hands, he clutched a novel he had not even bothered to open on the boat: Alberto Moravia's *The Empty Canvas*. At the age he was then, he was an empty canvas and no doubt in his still juvenile mind he found the book particularly appropriate. A hotel room in the Rue Saint-André-des-Arts was waiting for him. He was tired and needed sleep, but in his excitement, he could not sleep, and he knew he had to go out and walk. What he did or where he went was unavailable to memory. He imagined, writer that he was, that he would have strolled up the Boulevard Saint-Michel and then along the Boulevard Saint-Germain where he would have paused to look at Les Deux Magots and the Café de Flore. But all this was pure conjecture, and his mind dismissed the fiction of inventing it.

Then a door opened, and he was in a room. A naked man was in the bed. In his bed. It was no longer 1979, but the January of 1980 and he had already begun to teach English at that esoteric school whose main influences were the teachings of Rudolf Steiner. The naked man on the bed was Thomas. He was slightly older than Alex, and his chest was covered in soft, blond hair. He had cuddled against this man, but they had not had sex, of this, he was sure.

"Why can't I do anything with you," Thomas asked.

"I just can't respond."

"Don't you find me attractive?"

The usual cry of vanity.

Alex saw the wallpaper. It was busy and bucolic: a countryside scene repeated over and over, covering all four walls of the room—a young woman bending over, pouring milk into a jug, and nearby, a young man watching. He wanted to get out of the room. The repetition of this motion of milk and jug oppressed him.

"We can go out for dinner and talk," Thomas suggested.

Alex replied that he was not free as he had a private lesson to give.

"I'm sorry," Thomas said, and his golden body leapt out of bed and hurriedly dressed. Alex looked in fear at the body and how it had wanted to press into his own, penetrate him with endearing words. Why he was afraid, memory now would not tell him.

Alex's mind was racing, busy weaving the fiction that he would want to call the truth.

He was in the classroom where a group of students, mainly women, were watching him as he made them repeat English words. It was a small, stuffy and dismal room in a big house near the Luxembourg Gardens. He could no longer name the street or recall details of the interior, only the bleak impression of dullness and lack of interest in the room. Why did they bother to attend his classes when it was apparent none of them wanted to? But that was not entirely true. There was a woman in her seventies, Jacqueline, she did want to learn, and on several occasions, she invited him to her flat on the Rue Bonaparte. It was there in that room, knowing that the school would be closed for July and August, that she offered him a temporary job near Bordeaux teaching two boys whose mother was a friend of hers.

"But I had planned to go back to England this summer."

"Is that what you want to do?"

"My parents are getting on, and although they dislike me, I feel it is my duty to go." The words had been said, and the memory hit him with full force. They disliked him.

"Nobody dislikes their children," Jacqueline said.

"They did not want children. I was an accident," he clarified, "but they still support me financially, enough to live here. What I earn at the school gives me just a bit extra."

"Dislike from one's parents. It's appalling, like something out of Dickens," she cried and raised both hands in the air. Alex remembered her face clearly. How old she had appeared to him then. "It is a house in the countryside," she persisted. "Set in its own grounds. A car will meet you at Bordeaux. The children are around eleven years old and a bit difficult, but their mother says that with the right person, they will be good."

Fiction created this dialogue, but it was more or less as he remembered. He wrote to his parents about the summer job, and they approved. The day he boarded the train, his heart was heavy. He did not get on well with children. He pictured two nasty little boys playing tricks on him, and to soothe his mind, he wrote a short story. It was a pale imitation of *The Turn of the Screw* and was full of clichés, ghosts, and people screaming in the night. He had almost finished it when the train drew into the station.

The rest is lost. There was no way Alex could retrieve his reasons for leaving the family, nor the cold way they had responded to his decision. On his return to Paris, Jacqueline was so cross with him that their friendship had ended. Alex remembered her looking at him sternly.

"You made me look foolish," she said.

"I am sorry."

"It's not enough. They have written to me and said you were ill-chosen, and that I was responsible. And I *am* responsible. I was responsible for believing in you. You have to grow up," she said finally, and closed the door.

Jean-Paul Sartre is dead, was all that he could remember thinking as he stood alone looking up at the iconic spire of Saint-Germain-des-Prés. It was a thought that crashed into his mind. The great man is dead. What of the Café de Flore now? How will it continue to exist? These foolish questions had, of course, no answer, except that as the months and soon the years passed, he saw that the Café de Flore did very well. It became a habit for him to frequent the place, reading upstairs and watching the parade of good, and not so good-looking men come and go. He went off with a few of them, and the impotence he had experienced with Thomas went away, but it was not the sort of sex he wanted. He told himself he was being used and he attempted to wrap inaccessibility around him like a cloak. In his one-room flat in the Rue Severo, he would wash himself each night with cold water, and only when the sexual need grew too insistent did he relieve himself of desire.

Was it 1981 or 1982 when he left the school and found another in the ninth arrondissement? Alex thought it must have been 1982. Paris was his home now, he told himself. The school was in a street he could no longer locate in his mind, but he recalled the nearby dry garden with its statue where he would routinely eat his lunch. It was in a nearby bookshop that he found a Livre de Poche of *Le Grand Meaulnes*. He read it quickly and with passion, and immediately read it all over again. He wanted to catch a train to the Sologne to try to find the places mentioned in the book and perhaps others that were not mentioned, but he never did. The days and months passed, and he grew bored and tired.

Alex was uncovering more memory than he thought he would. Two ugly encounters were lurking in his mind like monsters about to break down a door. He held them at bay with the misguided but insistent thoughts of purity and innocence he had had back then. Put simply, he needed, and *need* was the word, to find that young man who would be the equivalent of Yvonne de Galais in the book. He was no Meaulnes. He knew that. But he was, in essence, a wanderer and a loner. He no longer mixed with people, except of course those at school, but after that, no one. He had no friends, and he told himself he had no need for friends. He blamed the French partly for this, labelling them distant and arrogant, when it was he who was arrogant and enjoyed being apart. He was conservative in his clothes and avoided places where he would have to mix with young people or hear popular songs, especially English ones. He disliked the music of the time, and when in class he was asked by a young woman what he listened to, he was taken off guard and replied, "I do not have any records."

Her name was Martine. He could see her now. A tall blonde with large breasts and a loud voice that hit him like a verbal whip.

"Depeche Mode. What do you think of them? Have you heard Alison Moyet, and can you name any of the songs from *Upstairs at Eric's* by Yazoo?"

"No, I've not heard them," he replied.

"When she sings *Goodbye Seventies* it's like an anthem that we must move on."

Alex imagined as he recalled this encounter that he told her to return to learning the rules of English grammar, but he could still see that look of cold contempt in her eyes that said quite clearly in French, *pauvre con*. He realised very well then that he had been born to be disliked, and that the source of this *was* his parents.

A young man in the class joined forces with Martine to sneer at him. He recalled the day when this youth, whose name was Benoît got up, tore up his exercise book and walked out of the room.

"You are an old man already," Benoît hissed in English before slamming the door. Martine sniggered in her seat, but when he asked her to recite a poem from Byron without looking at her book, she got to her feet and in near-perfect English went through *When We Two Parted*.

It was that day (and this he was sure was not fiction) that he bought Julien Green's *Moira*, and along with *Le Grand Meaulnes,* it became his obsessive read. He identified with Joseph Day, and except for not having red hair, he saw a lot of that character's nature in him. When the head of the school asked him who were his favourite authors, in cold reply, Alex replied, Alain Fournier and Julien Green.

"What dismal choices," the elderly master replied, looking him up and down, and no doubt questioning why he had employed him. "Don't you have any favourite English authors? After all, you are English, aren't you?"

Alex said nothing.

"No one comes to mind?"

Alex could not recall exactly how he had replied, but he thought he had said, "Emily Brontë and Thomas Hardy."

"And why do you have a fondness for these writers?"

"I have no idea."

"Well, that seems strange to me. Neither are particularly interesting to me, but at least you seem to know them."

"I can assure you, Monsieur, that I have read them."

"What about the moderns? What about Iris Murdoch or Ian McEwan?"

The rest of the questioning, Alex had lost somewhere deep in the depths of himself. All he knew was that the man held him in as much contempt as most of the class.

It was a year later in 1984 that he began to explore the Marais and discovered Les Mots à la Bouche bookshop: an Aladdin's cave of gay books and images. He was excited by the magazines with semi-naked men on their covers, and like Joseph Day in *Moira* he at first ran from such temptation, but the urge for sex nagged at him like a bad tooth causing pain and demanding attention. He bought a copy of *Querelle de Brest* and left the shop. He sat for a while in the Bar Hotel Central next door and drank more wine than he was used to. Several men approached him, and one of them did interest him, but not enough. He left the quartier and walked towards the Seine. It was a beautiful day, or if it wasn't, it should have been, and Alex let the fiction say that he found a seat on the quai and read Genet for a full four hours. This book revealed a new world for him. There was nothing of the pleading and begging for acknowledgement he had come across in American and English gay literature. Nor did the book deal with Aids which, as he had kept himself away from gay life for so long, Alex felt had no real relevance to him. The buggering of Querelle in the book stirred him to an erection, and he walked to the nearest café, just behind the BHV department store, to sexually relieve himself with almost painful urgency. Afterwards, he returned to the same bench by the Seine and continued to read. A man in his late thirties or early forties sat next to him and glanced at the book. Alex was so engrossed that he did not notice. It seemed as if the man had come from nowhere.

"Genet!" the man exclaimed, and Alex turned his head to look at him. He had rugged features: blond with reddish skin, and deeply inset blue eyes. Alex desired him, but feared the man was somehow incompatible with him. "I read Genet years ago," the man said as if responding to a question.

"Did you like him?"

"Very much. Have you read *Pompes funèbres*?"

"No, this is the first book of his that I've read."

"I suggest you read *Pompes funèbres* next. Your accent is English?"

"I am English."

"London?"

"No, Brighton."

Alex refused to recall any more of this trivial conversation. He had been approached by this man, and he had been questioned about Genet, but he was generating a false memory by attempting to reproduce the exact dialogue. He neither wanted nor had to create any fiction about this encounter with Loïc. He recalled the name out of so many that he had forgotten and had no idea why; its singularity perhaps, as he had never encountered a Loïc before or since. He had no desire to ask the man about its origins as he had no real desire to go further with him, and yet further he went.

They took a taxi at Châtelet and ended up at a house in Auteuil.

"My wife has just died."

These words had remained firmly within Alex, close to his consciousness, and once recalling them, he recalled the rest of the words that were said. Alex, or the Alex he did not know within himself, allowed them to come to the forefront of his mind.

"She died of cancer. I watched the end. I am still in shock."

"Then why are you with me?" Alex asked.

"Because I like young men as well as women. Usually when I choose a woman, she is older than me. I like women in their fifties. I am attracted to their bodies at that age and to their experience of life. My wife died when she was sixty. We had been together for eight years. During that time, I never once went with a man. You are the first."

Alex was silent. He lay in the vast bed looking through the tall windows to a garden filled with statues in the distance. He did not ask him why he was not attracted to men of his own age. That knowledge seemed futile. The whole experience of sex with this man had been futile. Alex had been quickly turned over on his stomach and then fiercely penetrated. It was painful, and Loïc had taken a long time to reach his climax. Alex decided he would never see this man again, but that promise to himself proved to be false. He saw Loïc often, and the more he saw him, the more he desired his body and enjoyed showing him what he, Alex, liked to do in bed. This precarious relationship lasted for nearly six months, and they met regularly twice a week. Loïc had habits. They always met at Châtelet and always took the same route by taxi. If the taxi driver deviated, he was promptly told to return to the original route. Only once did a driver refuse to do this.

"I know the route," the taxi driver had insisted.

"But it is not *my* route," Loïc had angrily replied. "I am paying you to take me the way I want to be taken; to approach my house in the way that I want to approach it. Is that understood?"

"I do not like to be told how to do my job. My way is shorter, and you pay less money. Isn't that attractive to you?"

"I'm not poor," Loïc had arrogantly replied. "I will not pay you at all if you don't go back and follow my instructions."

"Alright, I get the picture. You want total control. I'm glad you are rich enough to always get your own way." The taxi driver gave in to him, reversed the car and submitted to the dogmatic core of his temporary master.

All the time that Alex was seeing Loïc, he had never once asked him about his profession, and Loïc behaved similarly. When they did talk, it was not about past relationships (no more was mentioned of his recently deceased wife), only about books, music and theatre. He had to be the master in what he chose to talk about. Neither of them was in love with the other or even approaching that mysterious state. Loïc's taste in the arts was classical, and the borders of their conversation were as precise as those in the garden, where the statues of naked men and women were arranged with mathematical precision, in stark contrast to the wild and romantic gardens that Alex recalled from England.

Seated on a bench one evening, although it was winter and the sky was darkening, Loïc announced, "I think we have exhausted each other."

"Yes," Alex replied simply.

"It was good, but we have gone as far as we can go."

Not being able to resist, Alex added, "We have followed the same route too often. That is exhausting in itself."

Loïc did not reply to this, but Alex noticed him straighten up on the seat. Whatever he felt about such a barbed remark, he was not going to comment on it.

Alex had to find his own way back from Auteuil and choosing not to take a taxi he decided to walk. There had been no goodbyes, just the opening of a door, a clasp of hands as if some business had been concluded, and then Alex was alone outside. During the time they had seen each other, Loïc had never explained why, with all his money, he did not have a car. One final mystery; at their first encounter, Loïc had recommended Genet's *Pompes funèbres,* but among his vast library, Alex had not seen a single book that related to the twentieth century. As he walked back into the centre of the city, Genet's title *Pompes funèbres* came back to him again and again. He left, without animosity (was that true?), thrown out like a corpse and without much ceremony.

Alex felt soiled by this almost relationship and vowed to never embark on another. Such was the naive thinking of a bruised young man, and in his way, Alex had been bruised by Loïc. The words about *exhausting* each other seemed cruel in retrospect, and yet paradoxically (masochistically?) he respected Loïc's clarity. He realised the French were experts in it and that they knew exactly where to place the invisible knife: the blade that had scraped some skin from Alex's flesh.

He continued giving private English lessons, but despite some pupils' attempts to reach him as a person, either emotionally or intellectually, he always kept them at arm's length. It was during this period that Alex wrote his first novel. He even found an English publisher for it. The few reviews that appeared in the press said that he showed promise, but that the characters were lifeless and needed more experience, or at least some knowledge of themselves. Rereading the book many years later, Alex agreed. His three main characters had no inner lives. The next was better, but it was after his relationship with Luc that he opened up as a writer.

It was 1985, and he was still in Paris. He went out rarely, and his many pupils took up much of his time. As for his sexual life, he made use of cabins in sex shops and watched a lot of pornographic films, but more often than not, he left the cabins without achieving a climax.

The only area of Paris he liked to visit was Montmartre. He enjoyed the fakery that epitomised the quartier and being among tourists even though he considered himself to be by now a Parisian. He would get off the Metro at Anvers, climb the hill lined with shops full of trinkets and gaudy souvenirs and then take the funicular up to his destination. He never entered the church but would stand for hours against the balustrade and survey the city and its landmarks below. After that, he would return home. He had seen Paris: the Paris that he needed so much, and he had held it like he held humanity, at a respectful distance.

Looking back and analysing both the fiction and the reality of all this, Alex realised that not once during that year had he taken on the Aids crisis that surrounded him. It was at the back of his mind, of that he was sure, but it was never brought to the front. Loïc had always used a condom, as had Alex when the sexual roles were reversed, and since then, he had not had sex with any men. The wall, for wall it was that closed him in, also protected him from awareness. He dismissed any notion of existential *bad faith*. It was an accident—an accident in the street that jolted him back to some sort of connection with others.

It was night. He was walking through the dark streets of the Marais, near Saint-Paul, and ahead of him was a young man on a bike. Suddenly, from a side street, a speeding car crashed into the bike, and the young man was crushed under its speeding wheels. The vehicle continued without stopping, and Alex was alone with the prone figure in the street and the tangled mess of the bicycle. The young man was bleeding profusely and went into a convulsion, twisting around as if to attain some impossible escape from his condition. He then died on the tarmac. All the pent-up emotions inside Alex came to the surface. He cried, bent over the body and then let out a howl for help. A light came on in a nearby house, and soon there were a few people and then a crowd, all surrounding this once vital man, now contorted in his last agony. None of them were aware that it was Alex who had screamed so violently, and he could not face giving evidence either to the ambulance that had been called, or the police. He had not been able to take the car's number, and as Paris was full of black cars, he knew well enough that whoever was responsible would probably get away with their crime. He protected himself by slipping away, but he was changed. The shock of what he had seen burnt into him, and he suffered with an intermittent fever for a couple of weeks. Over and over in his nightmares, he saw the young man's final moments and his attempts to twist away from the inevitable. He had seen death. Even after the fever had gone, he remained mainly in his apartment, only going occasionally to a corner shop to get essential food. He lived on packet soup, bread, and a few biscuits, and drank water from the tap. During those long days and nights, he thought of death constantly, and came to the conclusion that all young men must, and that he too would die. I could not save him, he thought to himself. I could not keep him alive. Why should I live? Why should I, a coward who was too frightened to remain at the scene to give evidence, survive?

Three weeks later he went to a gay sex cinema and had sex with an unknown man without a condom. He had taken condoms with him, and had intended to use them, but when the moment came, the man knocked the condom out of his hand, bent him over and fucked him. Afterwards, he went into a rundown toilet in a café nearby and noticed that he was bleeding. He washed himself as best he could and went home. Had he gone there with the condoms intending for this to happen? Over the years, he thought again and again of the motivations, mainly hidden, that had led him to that encounter. There was a contradiction he could not solve. He had taken condoms, so surely he had not wanted it to happen. But the inner self can be perverse, and maybe the condoms were a false mascot held to conceal his real intentions.

Real intentions? Alex paused in his reflections. His remembrance of what had happened was perhaps a fiction. Was his mind now telling him that the condoms existed and hiding the truth that he had gone to the cinema without them? It was too far back, too far back and covered with so many layers of time. He had to be honest and admit to himself that the exact truth could not be excavated and brought into the light.

His mind jumped to the first months of 1986. He had to confront his first meeting with Luc. All else was of no importance: the way people looked or lived, and how many deaths there had been because of the virus. He went to Les Mots à la Bouche often and bought new books that appealed to him. The titles eluded him, as it was still mainly *Le Grand Meaulnes*, *Moira*, and his bible *Fabrizio Lupo* that he read and re-read. They kept him sane in what was an insane period. He still had a longing to go to the Sologne. The mystery of the place filled his mind with comfort as if it was there or a place accessible to there that he would eventually find his home. It was one night after finishing *Fabrizio Lupo* and looking again at a few pages of *Le Grand Meaulnes*, and in a mood of high romanticism that he returned to the same cinema he had been to before. Why was this romantic? His two favourite books had left him excited for contact. He needed, had to touch, another body. He found a man he liked and had sex with him, and this time he did use a condom but after he withdrew he saw that the condom was no longer there. He assumed as the place was dark that the condom had fallen off upon withdrawal, and he dismissed all thoughts of danger. I protected myself, he thought as he walked away from the cinema. Despite remaining apart from others, he had begun to seriously long for just one person; one person who would reach the coldness he had built up over the years and burn it away. Alex paused. Is this all of the truth, he asked himself. There was a vast space between 1986 and 2020 in which a lot else had occurred, burying precise memory of those months. Why, why had the force of Luc returned to him at Ned's place? What was the point of trying to probe, to recall, to re-experience, or perhaps to excuse himself? For a while, he closed the book within him: the book of a long-lost experience that had been the most painful as well as the most beautiful of his life. He paced the room, needing sleep, but a voice inside him was saying, I am here. I am here. Remember me. The voice was quiet but insistent, and then he saw a vivid image of Luc holding up the Alain Fournier book. Such dreams, the voice continued, and you will never know if I am alive or dead. Alex cried out, and the image and the voice disappeared. He had been called to remember and remember he must, as much of the truth as possible; no flirting with lies or nostalgia for a lost idyll. He went over to the Livre de Poche of *Le Grand Meaulnes* and found that it was breaking apart at the spine. He did not dare open it lest it fell apart, and he turned instead to his Penguin edition: *The Lost Estate*. The title was good, and it reinforced to Alex that he too had lost the estate of the young man he had so wantonly abused, and that included himself as well as Luc. "Look the truth straight in the face," he said to himself. "You can never, ever go back. No amount of recall can do that. Time is moving on, and somehow this night has to be a penitence for what happened; for what you and Luc lost in your estate of being men." He knelt on the floor for a while and placed his hands in prayer although there was no belief in God or eternal life within him.

He was, in fact, praying to the invisible presence of Luc inside him.

The day after the night at the sex cinema, I met him. Luc. I had been at the Café de Flore and decided to go and browse through the books at La Hune. I'm afraid of remembering him as being more beautiful than he was. I have to go easy with memory, draw it up slowly and with care. He was standing inside at the front of the bookshop glancing at the covers on display. One white row of new titles after another. He was engrossed, and yet paradoxically seemed distant from the books in front of him, as if none had any meaning. He did not notice me, and I had time to take in his looks; the way he stood and the way he would tentatively reach down and touch one of the books, and then hesitantly trace his fingers over another. He was slim and not very tall. His hair was light brown, his eyes grey. He had a fragility about him that I associated with tenderness, and that was the deepest impression I had of him: a tenderness of beauty. Alex thought all this to himself in this vigil of a night, forcing open the doors of recall to see once again what he had seen then. He did not want Luc to be a ghost of the past, but actually there, and for La Hune to be actually there, but sadly he realised that like La Hune, which no longer existed, it was possible Luc was no longer alive. Alex wanted to return to that bookshop one last time, to go up to that young man and say, "Forgive me. Can you ever forgive me?" But time, the invisible enemy that draws us inevitably forward, forbade such an act, and only in the mirror of memory could he see Luc again.

He stood beside him and picked up a book. His vision was blurred as if a sudden and brutal tiredness had impaired it. All of literature was meaningless to him, even his own.

"There's not much of interest here, is there?"

Luc stared at Alex, and Alex saw how big his eyes were in contrast to the rest of his face. His skin was pale, and as he spoke, he brushed his hair back away from his forehead. Yes, that is exactly what happened. Alex had no need to elaborate or to create a romantic fiction about it. He had to know him, had to see him again, and even if they did not make love, it would be alright. He just wanted the privilege of being near him. For a moment, nothing more was said. Luc continued staring at him, and Alex had the impression that he knew exactly what Alex was feeling.

"Do you come to this bookshop often?" Luc asked.

"Yes," Alex replied.

"I'm surprised we have not seen each other before. I live in the Rue du Bac. I came in for a specific book today, but first I wanted to look here. It's always intriguing to see how much commercial rubbish is being produced."

"I live on the other side of the river. Near the Rue Rambuteau."

"But you like Saint-German? The boulevard? The life here?"

"Yes, I like it. What book did you come in for?"

Luc smiled for the first time. He had a broad smile and small, perfect teeth. A few lines creased his face, and Alex knew that perhaps he was older than he looked. He had imagined him, at first sight, to be in his very early twenties.

"Oh, something very old. Very, how shall I put it, unfashionable? Goethe's *Elective Affinities*."

"Have you asked them if they have it?"

"No, but I expect they do. They have a good German section, and ideally I would like to read it in German."

"I am English, and I only read and speak French, but I share your liking for Goethe and other German writers, Novalis for instance."

"Also a great writer," Luc said, and his face became serious, and the lines disappeared.

Alex then dared to suggest, "Maybe we could talk over a drink. I was in the Flore earlier." Nervously, he waited for a reply, dreading that the answer would be a polite no, but Luc avoided answering and simply moved away from Alex towards the German section. Alex followed and saw him bend down to a lower shelf.

"I have found it!" he exclaimed. "And in German, what luck! You see, stupidly, I lost my copy on the Metro. I'm not usually careless. I have no idea how it happened."

"A thoughtless moment. We all have them."

Luc straightened up and held the volume of Goethe close to him. "Some people find this a difficult work to read. I have read it many times, and it has still not revealed all its secrets."

"The best books don't," Alex replied, but it seemed to him that his words were banal and lazily said. What he wanted to know was whether Luc would have a drink with him.

Now memory was going too fast. I did not even know his name at this stage, he thought. Alex went over to his bookshelves and picked out his Penguin copy of the book (He never really considered it a novel.) and looked at the Caspar David Friedrich painting on the cover. He kissed it and with that gesture, Luc, and La Hune, disappeared. He was conscious again of being in 2020. The gap between himself and that momentous day widened, and he could not go back to it in his mind. All he knew was they had told each other their names, and that they had had a drink in the Café de Flore, but downstairs. What they talked about was lost to him. The only detail that surfaced was a nearby restaurant where they had had a meal. It was not expensive, and Luc had paid for the meal. Had Alex proposed paying his share, or had Luc just taken control and considered it his place to do so? There was so much; so much deep down inside that Alex could not get to. He wandered around his front room and stared dismally at the pitch-black Brighton street outside, longing with intensity to be in France.

"Do you like Paris?"

More words returned.

"I live more or less—how shall I put it—a reclusive life. I like Paris very much, but I have this irrational fear that one day it will drive me away."

"You should not have such thoughts. Come back to my

apartment. I have a special wine you might like."

The dialogue ended there, and Alex struggled to recall the flat and the objects that surrounded Luc. He knew that Luc worked for a law firm, and this had surprised him as somehow, it did not seem to fit. He could not see him immersed in legal documents. Then he remembered. The flat was piled high with books, and there were many original paintings on the walls; all bought, Luc had said, from artists who would never have made a great success of their work. Mostly they were non-figurative, except for a small charcoal work of a naked man. Alex asked where he had bought it.

"From a *bouquiniste* along the Seine. An attic clear-out. It has no signature, but the faintness of the image appeals to me. He is walking, and he is naked, and at the same time, he seems on the point of disappearing."

Alex looked closely. It was true, the figure appeared to dissolve and fade into the background, grey on grey. He turned away from the drawing. Luc was standing very close to him. Oh, recall it all, recall it all, even if fiction has to come into it, and you have to give in to the lies of remembrance. Yes, Luc was very, very close, and their bodies touched. It was not Alex who made the first move, but Luc, who bent forward and lightly kissed him on the lips. It was the hesitation of intimacy that aroused Alex; the tenderness that he had perceived in Luc's character in La Hune. Luc wanted him, and once more he took control. They clung to each other, heat into heat. What words passed their lips were simple murmurings of pleasure. Alex felt he had found *the* person: his Yvonne de Galais, and although he was slightly taller than Luc, he sensed that Luc was the stronger. There was nothing soft about his slender body, and beneath the light shirt he was wearing, he felt tight flesh and a body waiting to give. The bedroom door was opened, and in the semi-darkness, they undressed and lay side by side on the bed. Their kisses lasted a long while, and Alex lay back as Luc slowly folded him into a firmer embrace. Alex knew that Luc wanted to enter him, and with gentle touches and a long and continually caressing prelude, he gave himself to him. There was nothing imperfect in the act; no fumbling or hesitation, simply a letting go on both sides. Alex thought, it has never been like this. It will never be like this again.

"I am happy," Luc said afterwards. "Talking with you in the Flore, eating together afterwards—I looked at you and knew that this had to happen, even if only once. It had to happen as if it were meant to be. I was not looking for a lover, but what happened just now, it was an act of love for me. No other act is possible."

"I know," Alex said. He then talked about his love for Alain Fournier's book, and Luc replied that he too had read it many times as he had been born in the Sologne.

Alex attempted to correct himself as he drew all this to the surface. Was there meaning in that first act of love? He wondered at the truth that was comforting him even now. Wasn't it during their second meeting that these words about Fournier's novel and Luc's birth in the Sologne had been spoken? Wasn't he merging these two encounters together? Hadn't Luc been more reticent in his words during their first, and more open about himself in the second. Some of what he now remembered was said that night, but wasn't their next love-making closer to a truth of love? He could not be sure. The only truths that were secure were that Luc wanted a sincere lover, that he loved the Fournier book almost as much as he loved Alex, and that he wanted sexuality to be a profound experience and not a superficial encounter. This was made clear in his words: *no other act is possible.*

It was during the third week of their relationship that Alex asked him what he had meant by these words.

"I'm afraid above all of meeting the wrong person for me," Luc replied. "I've gone with very few people. Something about you made me choose you, and I feel it was the same for you. I do not go into the homosexual milieu much, and I do not regret my choice to keep away from those places. I am aware of Aids, but I sense, perhaps foolishly, that it will touch neither of us. You are clean of heart, Alex, and I suspect you are also clean of body. I feel I have done all I can to prepare myself for the right person."

"How can you be so sure I am the right person?"

Luc sighed and said, "I am not a romantic. Contrary to the words I am using, I am very realistic about what I sense in others. I have often been told that I live in a world of fantasy, but it is not fantasy to me. You are not the personification of my dream of an ideal, but a reality in flesh and spirit that is solid and real. I fear the feelings of love that I feel."

"Why?" Alex asked.

"Because I dread betrayal more than anything else. And inevitable though I feel our meeting was, it was just the beginning of an awareness that we *could* mean everything to each other. Take my work in law, for example. I have to judge every case. I have to take time to grasp what has really occurred. I have to weigh up the possibilities of crimes and misdemeanours. Above all, I have to be conscious of lies, even when the person telling them believes them to be the truth."

"We make each other happy," Alex said.

"That's what I said when our relationship began. Perhaps I said it, and you did not hear it. I am happy. I said it was an act of love between us and I still feel that it was, but betrayal can split the memory of that act, and worse still, it can tear apart the inner reality of being in love."

"I want to say simply, I love you."

"So do I. I look at you, and I think, let the time come when it is said with total trust, and no possibility of betrayal."

"And that is not now?"

"Time has to pass. We will know when we have reached that point of absolute unity. Each act of love is part of creating the singleness that is us together. Each act of love is a foundation stone."

It was a month later. Luc had left Alex alone in the flat for a few days and, drawn by temptation, he opened Luc's writing desk. In a semi-hidden drawer, he found a small red notebook. Alex remembered how his hands had trembled. He was going to do something he had no right to do. He was going to read it. There was nothing much in the first few pages, but written very quickly, for he noticed how erratic the pen had been on the page, he read the words: *Can I trust him? Will he betray me like Bertrand?* He read on. The exact words were beyond faithful recall, but the essence was that Luc had had a previous relationship.

Alex paused in his journey through memory. He threw aside suddenly all he had thought about their first encounter, their second, and the weeks that followed. I am putting Luc up on a pedestal of purity, but he was not like that. I am lying. Cut out the romantic. For although he believed Luc had said those words to him, he was adding a gloss. It was the sort of fiction that he utterly dismissed; feel-good novels with high ideals that certain gay writers use to promote the best of homosexuality. It existed in heterosexual novels too. He thought of Françoise Sagan's *La Chamade*. She did not show her main female character in the best light, nor the males around her, but the concentration of ownership and desire within elitist Paris made the novel romantic. A state of sadness was achieved in the end because the heart had to say no. In his relationship with Luc, the heart did not have to say no. It was a social action that brought disaster to them, that caused heartbreak.

Sitting down at four in the morning, drinking coffee, he re-opened the red notebook.

Who had been Bertrand?

Luc had met him at a dinner party given by one of the lawyers. The older man in front of him at the table had a companion, and this young man was Bertrand. He was not much interested in law and was bored with the older man. Alex read on. The young man, Bertrand, was in clichéd terms a wolf in sheep's clothing. He latched on to Luc because he found him attractive. He arranged to meet him again, and a relationship began. What Luc later discovered was that he was one of Paris's most experienced male prostitutes, but what made him different was that he showed love for the money given and refused to acknowledge that he was selling himself. This duplicity of self is not uncommon, but Luc was not prepared for it. When he found out, he had a severe nervous breakdown. He couldn't eat. He lost weight, and like Alex, he shut himself away with his law books and concentrated solely on his job. He was only just emerging from this experience when he met Alex. It was all there in the red book. He also described the symptoms he had: his terror of people and how he could hardly bear to go near anyone and had to work from home in a lesser capacity than before. He had terrible nightmares and began to be afraid of disease and death. Night after night of waking up in a sweat made him fear he had contracted HIV. He got tested and was negative. This buoyed him up, but the possibility of death had put its seed firmly into his brain. He believed that all homosexuals would eventually succumb to the virus, and he sought refuge in old books and films in which no one was confronted with a pandemic virus. Then religion entered his mind, and he thought by living a clean and untouchable life that he would be saved from the horrors of an appalling death. He read *Le Grand Meaulnes* over and over, dreaming of his simple life in the Sologne and at the same time sharpening his mind in the pages of *Elective Affinities* and other philosophical works. In this way, he kept himself aloof from the fears inside him, but the fears remained nonetheless. He dreamed of having a clean relationship with a pure young man while waiting for the crisis of Aids to pass, which he feared might never happen. Towards the end of the notebook, further nightmares were mentioned, along with a terrifying nightly sensation that he was being throttled. After putting the notebook back in its place, Alex had one desire: to repress what he had read.

So far in his experience of sleeping with Luc, Alex had not

been awakened either by him having a night sweat or a nightmare, but one night, the dreams did return for Luc. Alex heard a howl, and woke to find Luc sitting up in bed, his body as cold as ice and shivering. He screamed loudly, and Alex held him close, both warming him and calming him down. Luc clung to him, and then with extreme force pushed Alex face downwards on the bed, and before Alex could stop him, feverishly penetrated his body. In a few minutes, the experience was over, and he had ejaculated inside him. The morning came and, for a while, Alex thought he had dreamt it all. Luc asked if they could do something special that day. He appeared to remember nothing of the night before.

"What do you suggest?" Alex asked.

"Let's get on a train and go to Orléans for the day."

Alex said that he had not been there before, and once on the train, Luc leant back in his seat and sighed. It was a sigh of relief.

"Tell me what you are thinking, Luc?"

"Oh, of Sologne and where I spent my childhood. Orléans is on the edge of it. Vierzon is further south. Perhaps one weekend in the future I will take you there."

The sky was cloudless, and it was a day of total happiness. Alex was happy because Luc was happy, and he felt closer to him than he had before. They visited the cathedral. The Loire was peaceful, and its waters flowed gently. The world seemed utterly at peace with itself. As night fell, they returned to Paris. It was only later that Alex admitted to himself he had felt uneasy with the smugness of the place and that the happiness he had felt that day had come only from Luc.

Time passed, and after several months Luc announced, "I feel we have reached that singleness of being. I love you totally."

"Are you sure?"

"I'm twenty-eight-years-old. I know. I'm sure."

"I love you as well," Alex replied, and deeply and sincerely, he felt that it was true.

That night, after these declarations, Luc awoke screaming, with tears pouring down his cheeks. "Help me," he cried out.

Alex turned on the light.

"I am here, Luc. It's alright, I am here."

"*Can* you help me?" the contorted face, aged by inner pain, cried back to Alex.

"You are safe. You are home."

"I dreamt I was in Hell. The place was burning, and there was no escape. A voice was repeating over and over, 'Homosexuals will burn forever.'"

"Hush, Luc, it was a nightmare. I have had equally bad ones."

"But is it true? Tell me, Alex."

"No, it's your mind playing at being the devil. There is no other place than this world, and after death, there is peace."

"Do you believe that?"

"Yes."

"Truly?"

"Yes, Luc, now settle back in my arms, and we will keep the light on for a while. There, put your head on my shoulder. I will be your refuge. I will whisper about places and things of beauty, and of the journey we are going to take to the Sologne. Soon you will drift off, and tomorrow you will forget all about this."

Luc fell asleep again, but Alex could not. He caressed the hair on Luc's head, and sat there until morning, watching his lover, fearful for him and his sanity. Clearly somewhere deep down, Luc was struggling with his sexual orientation.

The weeks passed and a routine set in. Luc had less bad nights, and his strength of mind returned to how it had been when they first met. They loved the cinema, and often they tracked down obscure films playing in the smaller cinemas that were dotted all over Paris. Returning home one night after seeing *Manon '70* with Catherine Deneuve, Alex ran a hot bath. The light bulb in the bathroom had been replaced with a much brighter one, and looking down at his body, Alex saw that his chest was covered with a rash. He knew something was wrong. He had also had headaches and muscle aches, but now he sensed that something serious was attacking him from within. He did not want to frighten Luc, and after putting on his clothes, he returned to the bedroom.

"Why are you dressed?" Luc asked.

"I feel cold. Maybe I've got a cold or flu. I'd better sleep on the couch in the living room."

Luc immediately got up, made up a bed for Alex on the sofa and found him a pair of pyjamas. "I'll make an appointment for you to see my doctor," he said.

While Luc made Alex a hot drink in the kitchen, Alex turned off the living room light and changed into the pyjamas.

"Why are you sitting in the dark?" Luc asked when he returned with the drink.

"It's just that the light hurts my eyes."

"You must definitely see my doctor tomorrow. I'll make an appointment first thing in the morning."

Alex tried but failed to block out the rest. He did not want to go deeper into memory, but he had to. It was syphilis. The doctor, who was a personal friend of Luc's, instructed Alex to inform him immediately. The cold way that Luc received the information was frightening, and equally frightening was the way he told Alex he would never forgive him and that he would never see him again. As he recalled their final parting, it was as if Alex had received a blow to the head, and no longer bearing the weight of his guilt, he crawled into bed. It was light now, outside in Brighton, and he shrank down into the folds of the sheets, his head still pounding. After all those years, he longed to hear Luc speak again; an ageing man now who perhaps would have the capacity to forgive. Closing his eyes, he remembered one last detail about those Paris days. Other than the night that Luc had penetrated him, there had been just two other times when, in their passion, no condoms had been used.

"There is no need," Luc had said. "We are clean."

Part Three
Separate people

Although he had not slept, Alex tried to brush away his thoughts of Luc. I must gain control of myself, he thought. I must not indulge in the Paris of the past, but if I do succeed in finding somewhere in France, it must be as close to the city as possible.

The near-total destruction of Notre-Dame the previous year had wounded him deeply. How could Paris exist without its heart? For centuries the cathedral had stood, and now the scaffolding, which was not even a part of the building itself, was threatening its survival. He had read that not until the spring or summer of 2020 would they know for sure whether the building could be saved or not. Maybe he was exaggerating what he had read, but even the remotest chance that the cathedral might disappear was unendurable. It was not only the centre of Paris, it was the heart of inspiration to all the other churches close by which like satellites revolved around it. This hurt him the most. He imagined Saint-Julien-le-Pauvre and Saint-Séverin looking towards the empty space where the solar force had existed, and he imagined the silent crying of the stones. His fantasy of the stones of those churches knowing that they were the children of the cathedral and weeping, was impossible. But what about within? It was as if they breathed, and surely if they breathed, then waters of loss could flow within and from them.

He had to do something, anything, to get rid of the images of both Luc and Notre-Dame as they had been; intact and glowing with eternal youth. He looked through his bookshelves and found a copy of the Alain Fournier novel. I will take this to Ned, he thought. I will hand it to him personally, not just leave it for him to find. He desired to see this good man: this man so unlike Alan; this man who would not pass him in the street without acknowledging him. But, he realised, the old do not exist for gay men, not really. Despite all the talk of embracing diversity, what younger man would genuinely want to embrace the flesh of an old body out of desire? A peck on the cheek or a hug perhaps, but otherwise the old were either non-existent, or grandfather figures to look up to and mentally leech from as Alan had done. Such is the fate, Alex thought, of old and wrinkled skin that nonetheless holds a wealth of memory and past life.

In the rain, he walked up St James's Street. It looked especially desolate in the grey morning light. Several tents, the only affordable places for those who had no homes, were pitched there, their occupants still dreaming in their hunger and their despair. Had Brighton a disproportionate number of them compared to other places? Either way, however many there were, it was a shame and a scar on the city. He recalled how a month before Christmas he had gone into a restaurant which had a tent pitched outside. The flaps were open, and inside he had glimpsed the pitiful possessions of a person who had nowhere else to go: dirty blankets and a few torn magazines, including of all things a Guardian travel supplement. This enraged him. He had to let off steam, to cry out against this brutality in the city's so-called heart.

"I want to speak to the manager," he had asserted. Several people seated at the tables eating, looked at him, and one man winked to another as if to say, "Here comes trouble."

The woman he had asked said, "What's it about? He's busy."

"Busy where?"

"Calm down," she whispered. "The whole place can hear you."

"Good."

"No, it's rude. You could at least keep a polite tone when you speak."

"I want to talk to him. It's urgent," he insisted.

"I asked you what about."

Her voice was prim, faked, and too classy for this second-rate restaurant. She wanted to be above him, to be superior. To Alex, at that moment, nothing seemed equal in Brighton.

"It's about the tent outside," he replied.

"Oh, that!"

"It isn't a that! It is a home. A home!" He was shouting now, and the manager as if by magic appeared beside her.

"What do you want?" he asked in a growl of anger.

"The tent. You must know it's there and that somebody lives there. You can see it."

"I don't watch it. I have better things to do. What about it? There are other shops and doorways down the street, also with tents. Why don't you pester them?"

"This is the only restaurant with a tent in front of it."

"So what?"

"I want to know if you ever give the person food."

"Don't be ridiculous."

A man, nearby, who had been listening, said, "You tell him, Marco."

Alex was insistent. "Not even leftovers? You must have leftovers in your kitchen."

The woman backed away, and her face turned pale. She pretended to get on with her work and prodded at a salad bowl.

"Waste food is disposed of in the proper way."

"You may call it proper, but I don't. Tell me, do you ever go out and ask whether the person is hungry? Do you know what that is? Hunger?" All around he could hear the sound of knives and forks being set down. The whole restaurant was now listening.

"Yes, as it happens, I do know what it is like," Marco said. "In Italy, I was hungry for months. No one gave *me* food."

"You have a cross around your neck."

Marco shrugged. "So?"

"A Christian cross."

"You got something against religion?"

"In many ways, yes, but the words of Christ have some meaning for me. It is a Christian thing to feed and give to the poor."

"Oh, go away," the woman at the salad bar said softly, and then returned to the kitchen.

Alex did not go away. He was hot with rage. He had to prove a point with this man; he had to express the injustice of it all.

"I am sorry no one in Italy gave you food, but that does not mean you have to behave in the same way. I just need to know if you ever think about going to that tent to ask. The offer may be refused, or it may be accepted. Don't you have a moral duty to help in some way?"

"I never complain about them being there; a man and a woman. I never tell them to shove off."

"Oh, go home!" a woman shouted from a far table.

Alex turned and looked at her. She looked bewildered by this and disturbed.

"It's all much ado about nothing, Cheryl," her female companion said.

"She's right," Marco said. "Leave my restaurant."

Alex felt he could not leave without forcing an answer to his question.

"Do you, or do you not, ever think of offering them food?"

"Do you want me to get help and push you out?"

"Do you ever offer?"

"No!"

The answer was shrieked back, and Marco momentarily had to steady himself against a pillar. Alex heard the answer, and with whistles of contempt from various tables, he left the restaurant. He had heard the voice of a Christian.

He had made his stand. He felt no pride in what he had done. He had seen the open void of the grimy tent, and he had seen a restaurant sign above it. He had simply wanted to know whether there had been any gestures of humanity from the restaurant, even once a day, a simple gesture in the land of the indifferent and the complacent. And at the same time as he exited, he questioned how much he helped the homeless. He gave money when he could, but the message from the authorities was that that was wrong. After all, the homeless may squander it on drugs or something inessential. Alex rejected this authoritarian position and believed that despite the food banks and the people who gave out free meals and shelter for the homeless, he should have the right to offer financial help and give *them* the choice to use it how they wanted. It was not an opinion widely held.

Ned was surprised when he answered the door dressed in a patterned pair of pyjamas with slippers on his feet.

"Oh, I thought you were the postman," he said. "I've only just got up. Had a rather bad night. I never like to meet handsome younger men like this. I would have got myself spruced up." He smiled his generous smile. "But now you must come in and have some coffee."

Alex said that he had come as promised with the book.

"So thoughtful, and so soon!" He took the book from Alex's offering hands. "And you have wrapped it in Christmas paper. I like that. It makes me think I'm getting lots of gifts. Anyway, it's freezing out here with the wind blowing."

"Maybe, we should have a coffee together later?" Alex suggested.

"A date! How exciting! Tell me what time and I will be there."

"There's a Starbucks down the road."

"Oh, no, not there. All those spluttering students—and we don't want to catch you know what, do we?"

"Okay, you name the place."

"Can you come back here at three this afternoon? I can never remember the name of the place where I have tea up the road. It's near to the flea-market."

"I'll come back here."

"How exciting!" Ned repeated and then with another smile added, "Just ring the bell, I'll be ready."

It was nine in the morning, and Alex returned to his flat, set the alarm and had a few hours' sleep. When he looked at his mobile phone, he saw a message from Paul. It read, "Want to see you. Ring you back. Hate texts." The *want* to see you, seemed more of a demand than a request. It was half-past two, and he had to go back to Ned's place. He had no time to shower, and simply put on an eau de Cologne he had bought in Paris.

"There you are," Ned said as he opened the door. He was smartly dressed in a grey suit with a grey overcoat and a bright yellow scarf. A striking combination, Alex thought. Yellow and grey go well together.

"Now, let me take you to my favourite café. It has the most delicious cakes, and I am paying!"

"Absolutely not," Alex replied.

"Look. I'm the one who declined the cheaper Starbucks, so it is my place to pay."

"I still say, absolutely not," and they both laughed.

The café was styled as shabby chic. An interior designer had done his or her best with miss-matched crockery and comfortable chairs that were all upholstered in different textures and colours. The place would not have been Alex's choice, but in they went. A group of schoolgirls were just about to leave. A schoolmistress was with them, and they glowed with the magic and charm of the well-off. Alex was glad they were leaving.

"Must be Roedean," Ned quipped as they trouped out.

"Or Brighton College," Alex replied, "out for a treat. Fourteen of them!"

"Well, this is a treat for me. I know that. Let's take the one table those amazons did not conquer."

They ordered tea, and Alex chose a carrot cake while Ned opted for a meringue.

"I've definitely made up my mind to leave this country,"

Alex said.

Ned wiped his mouth with a napkin and said, "You look tired. You look as if you have had a sleepless night."

"Yes. I couldn't get Luc, the young man I mentioned from Paris, out of my mind."

"When did you know him?"

"Back in '86."

"Aah!" Ned sighed. "One of the bad years."

"Yes, Ned, a very bad year indeed. I hurt him so badly. I tried all night to disentangle real memories from the ones I have fictionalised in my mind since then."

"It can't be done." Ned paused. "You know, I remember it was a bad year here, but I can't recall a single thing that I did or thought. I guess I just sailed against the blast of the wind and got through."

"You have the touch of a poet in that observation," Alex said.

"Flatterer. I never understood more than the most basic poetry. You know, like they used to write in birthday cards."

Alex smiled and said, "Well, those simple words spoke to many hearts."

"Often to mine, sadly, but none were true, and no one remembers my birthday anymore. Do birthday cards still have such verses?"

"I don't know, Ned. I think they've probably gone out of fashion. By the way, when is your birthday?"

"November 6th. Scorpio. And you?"

"June. Gemini."

"I like Geminis. But now, let's get down to serious things. Do you want to tell me about Luc?"

"Would you be angry if I didn't?"

"Of course not. But all the same, you've been wounded. I can't remember *what* I said last night, but I can see the wounds clearly now. You look handsome, but very, very exhausted, and it's not only to do with a lack of sleep. You are full of conflict. Once upon a time, I thought I was clairvoyant, but now I know I just *see*."

Alex looked at the décor around him, and yearned for an old Paris café, one that had kept its original character, but he knew that relatively few still existed.

"I wounded Luc," he said.

"Literally?"

"Yes, as it happens. Not with a blow or any kind of violent attack, but through loving him. He was, you see, the first person to crack open the shield that protected me from loving."

"Were you such an enclosed young man?"

"I hid within myself. I am a loner, Ned. It's too late for me to change now. I perceive everything as separation, not joining. In all fields of life."

Ned looked down at the ruins of his meringue as if surveying the fall of Troy, and he picked over what was left with his fork. "That's sad," he said quietly, "and yet you have someone waiting in the wings, so to speak. I sense that quite clearly. You will either discard him or accept him." Alex saw tears in Ned's eyes as he looked up and at him. "I would do anything to be your age, Alex. You still have choices."

"The only choice I need to make is to leave this country."

Ned got unexpectedly cross at this and raised his voice slightly. "Don't be a fool. Is Brexit really that important? After all, before 1973 or whenever it was, we still all had to be checked and get our passports stamped. One of my most ancient passports looks like a badge of honour—so many stamps, in and out, and each country had its own image, its own self, its own identity. I think the whole European Union should break apart. Let the Germans be German again, and the French, French."

"Please, Ned, let's not argue over it. I am a remainer, and I think we are doing a great wrong. Can we leave the subject at that?"

"I think it is ridiculous to be in this mess of a European Union. I never felt part of it when we were in it. But I will stop going on about the subject. We all have our political opinions, and those opinions will not stop us being friends."

There was an uneasy pause, and Alex reached out and grasped Ned's hand on the table.

"I am going there not only because of Brexit; I have an affinity with France. Call it my spiritual home."

"I felt that once about Greece, but I'm not packing up to go and live in Mykonos. I'm English, and I cannot be anything else."

"Neither can I. But I prefer to reside in my spiritual home."

Ned drank the last of the tea in his cup, and then asked, "But what of the beauty of this city? Forget all the cock-ups and the horrible messes the council have made. There is still beauty here: walking on the pier, for example, fair weather or foul. I like to hear the noise that aggressive channel makes when it's having a bad mood, and I also like to see it lying out flat, like a pond, at ease with itself. I look at the special light; the extraordinary light of the city. I am happy living in Kemp Town, despite the sordidness of St James's Street. And by the way, I can tell you, it was always like that, even when I was a child." He paused. "And the Clifton area? Have you ever seen such beautiful houses as Clifton Terrace or Powys Square, not to mention Sussex Square and Adelaide Crescent? They are absolute jewels! I am a Brightonian, and you are too. I can sense it in you. It is you. You just don't realise it. And say you do go to France, and sometimes visit Paris. It's a long time since you lived there, and if you did manage to find Luc again, what would you say?"

Alex felt faint. He had not eaten much, and his mind felt suddenly confused.

"I would tell him I was sorry," he said.

"What if you didn't hurt him as much as you say you did? What if he has forgiven and forgotten? You know nothing of the man since 1986. We are at the beginning of a new decade, 2020! A momentous year! And please, no paranoia over this wretched virus. They'll have a vaccine soon and if we have to go out with masks on, so be it."

"There are probably still traces of me, in his blood. They will always be there."

"What? You are really not being clear, Alex."

"I gave him syphilis," Alex replied, and the room began to spin around him. He clung on to the chair. "I must make it to the toilet, Ned. Tell me where it is."

Ned gave him directions, and in that cramped and old-fashioned toilet, Alex vomited. He thought it would never stop, but where had it come from? There was nothing in him. He leant against the dull and dirty-looking wall, and the awful sensation of spinning suddenly stopped. He flushed the toilet twice, then rinsed his mouth out with tap water. In the mirror, his face looked as grey as Ned's suit.

"Are you sure you're not ill?" Ned asked when Alex made his way back to the table. The two women behind the cake counter looked at him suspiciously. They clearly did not want anyone bringing sickness into their place. And who knows, maybe he had *it!* He knew exactly what they were thinking. In defiance, he sat down, called to one of them, and asked them to bring some more cakes and a pot of tea. Hesitantly, the woman acknowledged the request.

"*I* can't eat any more," Ned said.

"I'm empty, and I'm hungry. It's foolish, I know, but I must scoff a couple of cakes and fill myself up with tea."

"As long as you are not seriously ill."

"Really, Ned, I'm okay now, and I'm the one who's paying. I insisted before we entered the place, and I insist again."

Ned paused, and then asked with a certain wariness, "Is it true, what you said? What happened between you and Luc?"

"Would I lie?"

"Of course not, but Alex, these things happen. You didn't mean to harm him. I presume you did not know."

"No, I didn't know. I was green as grass. I didn't notice any chancre. I saw the tell-tale rash one evening as I was getting into a bath. After diagnosis, I told Luc at once."

"Maybe—just maybe, you did not infect him."

"I did. Without Luc knowing, I went back to the doctor, who was a friend of his. He knew we were a couple, and he told me. It may not have been ethical, but he did. Luc had it also."

"I see," Ned replied.

The cakes and the tea came. Alex looked at the choice with distaste, but it was food, and he believed he needed it. He gobbled it up, and he noticed Ned look around awkwardly. He was embarrassed. This was clearly not the sort of afternoon he had hoped for.

"I always seem to mess things up," Alex said, wiping his mouth with a napkin.

"Don't be ridiculous. You've messed nothing up at all. You should have come in and had breakfast with me this morning. I would have made you bacon and eggs."

Alex laughed. He had to. Ned would forgive him anything. He was, as he had said before, a good man. They are rare, and they forgive. And yet, all the same, he knew he had stained their new contact somehow. Ned would forgive, but he would not forget some of their dialogue or his gorging of the cakes. Nor would the women who ran the place and who had observed everything with merciless eyes. They would remember the gobbling and the slurping of the tea. Their private schoolgirls and regular customers never behaved like that, and why in heaven's name was Ned with him at all—Ned who was old and had such good manners and was usually alone and quiet. How strange for him to bring a friend with the manners of a dog. Oh no, they would not forget. They would remind Ned in unspoken cold looks, and they would never see him in the same light again.

Alex paid, and Ned had thanked him for it.

"Shall we go?" Ned asked.

As they walked back towards St. James's Street, Alex realised sadly they would not meet again. He would not be able to face Ned again. They arrived at Ned's flat and Ned said politely that he looked forward to their next meeting, but there was no firm invitation. Solitary people are excellent at keeping to themselves, Alex thought.

The following day, Paul rang him. Alex took time in answering as he could see who it was and wanted solitude to consider his plans for France, but the phone was insistent. It was seven in the morning.

"Alex, is that you?"

"You know it's me, why ask?"

"If you don't want to speak to me, I'll hang up."

Paul's voice sounded strange, and he seemed out of breath and afraid. He was in trouble and had turned to Alex. All this Alex knew without another word being spoken.

"Do you want to come over?"

"I am in—"

"Trouble?" Alex asked.

"No. It's just—well, yes I would like to see you and talk to you. The situation is—"

Alex interrupted him and asked if he could wait an hour as he needed a shower and to clear his head. He said he had slept badly, which was true, and that he'd had recurring dreams about death and dying.

"I'll come in two hours," Paul said, and rang off.

Alex made coffee, had his shower and took down an old Peregrine book—*The Novel in France*. He had no idea why, but the book relaxed him even though he disagreed with the author's evaluations of particular works. Eventually, tired of reading, he put down the book and saw by his watch that it was well past nine-thirty, and now he felt anxiety. Was Paul playing games with him? He tried once more to concentrate on the book, but his mind was not on it. He could not stop the anxiety. He had been reading the section on Proust, and as he put the book down, he realised that his thoughts were being drawn to Combray. He had spent a few hours the night before looking for a house he could afford and had found one in Eure-et-Loir: in Illiers-Combray, the village that had been the inspiration for Proust's Combray, and which had been renamed in his honour The house was run-down and needed renovating, but it had two bedrooms and two attics, one of which needed some serious attention, as did the wiring which dated back to before the war. Above all, he liked the fact that the interior had been untouched by the sort of modernisation that blemished so many English homes, and there were odd corners and antique wood panelling. The place intrigued him, and his instinct told him it could be a home. The mind often organises itself very well, and he sensed it was not for nothing that he had picked up the book and been reminded of the Proustian connection. He had given up on Paul and was about to go out to buy some food when the doorbell rang.

His first impression on seeing Paul was how old he looked. The downward lines on his face seemed deeper, and his eyes, which Alex found his best feature, looked dead. He was shabbily dressed, with torn jeans and a dreary sweater, scuffed shoes and a coat that was far too big for him. His hair fell lankly forward. Alex paused too long before letting him in, and Paul said very quietly, "It might be sunny, but I'm shivering here. It's cold."

Alex apologised and made way for him to enter the flat.

"I'm scared," Paul said.

"I gathered that from your voice on the phone."

"Do you mind if I have a shower?"

The request startled Alex and reminded him of Paul's first visit. He replied that of course he could, and that while he was having it, he would go and get some food because there was none left. "I think we both need a good breakfast," he said, the nervousness in his voice showing through.

"Don't worry, I'm not going to steal something and do a runner."

"I didn't mean—"

"Well, don't even begin to think it."

This stirred Alex's anger. He hated that anger. There had already been enough of it between Paul and himself.

"I don't want any more arguments," he said firmly, clenching his jaws tightly as he looked at Paul.

Paul looked down and mumbled, "I'm shit tired at the moment. I'm sorry, Alex."

Alex gathered his money and his coat and without another word, left the flat. It was an uncertain day with a strong wind that hurried the clouds across the sky. He looked towards the sea and saw dark clouds approaching. He did not want to get caught in a downpour. As Paul had said, the too-bright sun was cold. He bought what he needed, and when he re-entered the flat, he found Paul standing naked in the room. His body was more muscular than he had expected, and the bush of hair around his penis excited him. Paul just stood there, as if wanting to be looked at. His cock was uncut. Its tip peeked out from beneath the foreskin. There were long veins which, like the long lines on his face, fascinated Alex, and he could not resist staring. Then he apologised as if he had done something inappropriate. Paul pretended not to notice and reached out for his clothes which were scattered on the floor.

"Find what you need?" Paul asked, bending down to pick up his underwear and socks.

"What we both need," Alex joked. "I hope your stomach is as empty as mine. I bought everything that's bad for us. Bread for frying, bacon and eggs, and jam."

He busied himself and tried not to watch Paul as he continued dressing. He went into the kitchen and Paul joined him.

"I feel better now," Paul said. "I couldn't use the bathroom in the house where I live. There are too many people. There has been a sequence of birthdays the past few days and far too many guests. This morning I found a gob of spit on the toilet floor." He paused and shuffled his feet.

"Go on, Paul."

"I didn't realise it, but I am so scared of them around me—their proximity. I have my room, but they barge in, and I don't have any privacy, and there's a girl there who keeps trying to come on to me."

Alex looked at Paul and said simply, "Do you mean you are afraid one of them may have the virus?"

"I—"

"Don't hesitate to show your fear. I'm afraid too sometimes." Alex wondered how bad things would get with the virus and when it would end. He followed the news sporadically and had heard there were only fifteen beds in the whole country for those seriously ill with it. How he hated this government and its predecessors for their systematic devaluation of the Health Service, and their dubious motives for wanting to see an American style of medical provision. Fuck America to hell, he thought.

"I felt panic. Almost two days of it while they were partying. A couple of them coughing constantly, and that gob of spit on the toilet floor really got to me. My mind has been racing. I don't want to die in a bed in a room surrounded by people in masks. And I don't want to live among strangers who could give me the virus—maybe not now but eventually. I can't go around wiping every door clean before I touch it. I can't wash all the surfaces they touch. Fucking paranoia! I am getting paranoid. I know it will increase, and no one around me talks about it, or cares about prevention."

Alex nodded and continued preparing the breakfast. He piled both plates high with food and took out some burnt toast from the toaster.

"I always get toast wrong," he said casually.

"Can I lay the table?" Paul asked.

"Thanks. I'll hand you knives and forks."

There was a calmness suddenly between them, and Alex had the strange feeling that deep down, they knew each other very well. The illusion sustained him.

At the table and after they had eaten, Paul asked quietly,

"Can I come and live here? Just for a while until I find an inexpensive room somewhere. I know it's an intrusion, and that we may not get on, but you are the only person I can turn to, and I really don't want to go back to Hull."

Alex looked at Paul and said simply, "It wouldn't work."

"I promise, no quarrels. I know I can be an insensitive bastard. Always have been. I guess I was born on isolation row."

"What in Hell is that?" Alex asked.

"A place I imagine where some babies are born and put into isolation rooms—a whole row of small little rooms for babies who have to be set apart."

"What an odd fantasy."

"Been in my head since I was a kid."

"How did it start, this fantasy?"

"I don't know. I can't explain. You're a writer. You could probably explain it better than me. Anyway, I'll try. It's a sort of punishment place where doctors put the babies they think are going to be difficult as they grow up." Then Paul became animated with the subject. "They look at the new-born child and think if he or she mixes too closely with others, they will cause trouble, be a disturbance to society. It's like the doctors are psychiatrists and know. The babies are kept in isolation so long that they get used to it, and when they are given back to their parents, they are in total isolation within themselves."

"Paul, that's terrible. Since you were a kid, you really thought you were one of those babies?"

"I think you might be laughing at me, but yes, I really believe it."

"I'm not laughing, Paul. It's just, well let's say it's the first time I have heard such a fantastic idea—and in my life I have listened to many fantasies."

"I saw the smile on your face as I was talking to you." Paul got up from the table and paced the floor.

"Sit down again. Don't be so touchy. We all have different fantasies. There are some pretty terrible images inside of us.

It's stuff we all have. I know I wasn't wanted as a child. Were you?"

"Never asked them."

This was said with such childish helplessness that Alex thought, I can't refuse him. He is, in his way, an isolated child. He can come here.

"Please sit down, Paul. I can tell your head is spinning."

Paul came back to the table and sat down. He looked at the greasy plates in front of him and not at Alex.

"It's in my head now," Paul said. "A doctor, looking at me as a baby and seeing—my future. At school, I joined the others, but I kept my distance at the same time. I tried to be tough. I went in for all the sports even though I hated the bloody gymnasium—climbing ropes like a monkey and all that. I preferred to be in the open air, kicking a ball on the field. Football, yes, but not rugby. All that filth and mud and grabbing at each other."

"I didn't like it much either. I usually fell sick on games days."

There was a long silence, and Paul tentatively looked at Alex. "Please help."

Alex smiled at him and replied, "I still don't think it will work, but let's give it a try. Also, you know I'm intending to move to France. It will take months to bring it to fruition, but I'm determined to go. In fact, last night before going to sleep, I searched the internet and I think I found the house I would like. It would be just under two hours to get to Paris."

"Can't you give this shithole of a place another chance?"

"No, I can't," Alex replied. "I can't bear it here anymore. It's a visceral feeling. It's deadly to me, like this new virus is deadly to some people."

"I'll try to understand, Alex, and I want you to know that I'll give you the same amount of rent that I pay in the house where I am living now. I promise. I refuse to stay here without doing that."

"We'll see."

"No, it's a promise."

"Okay, Paul, if you say so. Now let's clean up these dishes. You can wash, and I'll wipe. How about that for starting to live under the same roof?"

"Fine," Paul said, and began to clear the table.

Alex knew he wouldn't accept one penny from Paul. He didn't care if Paul felt guilt or anger over this, he just wouldn't.

"Have you got much to bring from Moulsecoomb?" he asked.

Paul smiled and said, "What do you think? A bundle of stinking clothes, and a few things collected over the years. I have an old toy bear." He paused and then added, "I loved my grandmother. She gave it to me before she died. She used to hold it during the blitz attacks on Hull, and she swore the bear saved her house. Next door's house was hit. All killed." He paused, and his voice sounded shaky, and at the same time, he looked as if he was afraid of showing any emotion.

Alex did not want to be moved, but he was. He was glad Paul had been loved by someone. Unconditionally.

Paul reached out and touched Alex's arm. "Thank you," he said.

The day turned out to be surprisingly fine, with not a cloud in the sky. Alex asked if he could accompany Paul to Moulsecoomb to give him a hand with his things.

"No, I'd better go alone. I just hope they're all out. I'll leave what I owe and be out of the house quickly. Anyway, Moulsecoomb's quite far. You don't want to traipse all the way out there."

"I could wait in a taxi," Alex replied.

"I can't afford a taxi, and I don't want you to pay. Please don't insist." There was a note of warning in Paul's voice.

Paul left the flat soon after, and once alone, Alex looked around him. He saw how neat the place was and realised that it would probably not remain in that state for long. He sensed Paul was untidy, and if he was, he would not want to be reminded about it. His pride was a force to reckoned with, and Alex already knew they would argue and that there would be endless apologies. He pretended to himself that he was prepared for this and that despite their proximity, they could remain separate people. He had to be separate, he could not be involved, and at the same time, he visualised the bush of hair around Paul's penis, and saw himself kneeling in front of Paul and taking the hardening cock in his mouth. To ease away the thought, he watched some porn, but as usual, it took a long while to find the right guy to ejaculate to. He had to fix on just one man, and often he would not be that attractive. This time, it was someone in their late twenties or early thirties. In the scene, he had a younger man with him, but Alex paid no attention to him. He concentrated on the man he had chosen and was faithful to him until he came. Then he immediately turned off his computer, wiped away the weak sperm that had come out of him, and still feeling unclean, had another shower. He looked at his ageing flesh as the water splashed down, and hated it as if it did not belong to him. He recalled Paul's body and its slim but muscular form but dismissed the image and reached for a towel. "I will soon be sixty," he said aloud to himself. Then, going to a cupboard where there was a bottle of whisky, he poured himself a large glass. He sat on the sofa and drank it slowly, waiting for Paul to ring the bell. He imagined him holding his belongings, and perhaps there would be a smile on his face. He hoped for a relatively tranquil start to sharing the flat. The sofa folded out to a bed. Paul would have that, and despite Alex's double bed, Alex assured himself that whatever happened, the two of them would never share it. "I know what to do if I feel desire," he said, looking down at his computer.

It was a long wait. At seven-thirty that evening, Paul appeared at his door, and despite his need for a tranquil beginning, the first thing Alex did was reproach him.

"You could have called. I couldn't go out because I didn't want you to have to wait around outside. You don't have your own keys yet."

"Sorry," Paul mumbled and collapsed on the sofa that Alex had been sitting on. Alex picked up the suitcase standing in the middle of the room and shifted it into a discreet corner. It was quite heavy.

"You don't have to do that," Paul said.

"I just don't want to trip over it. Now, what do you feel like eating?"

"I've already eaten."

"Then I'll eat alone," Alex said, and immediately felt he had made a terrible mistake in accepting Paul into his small flat. While in the kitchen, he decided that for as long as Paul was living there, he would have to make his bedroom into a place where he could both sleep and work. It would mean moving both his bookshelves and his writing desk.

"You're not angry with me, are you?"

Paul came into the kitchen and hovered over Alex as he cut up the vegetables.

"Make yourself a drink while I am doing this," he said in reply.

"I don't want us to start off in a bad way. I was delayed. They caught me in the act of leaving and wanted to get another month's money off me. I didn't have it, and one of the guys there who dislikes me, threatened to keep my things if I didn't pay up. It was a nasty afternoon. Fortunately, two of the women stood up for me and said they trusted me."

"I said this morning I could go with you."

Alex cut his finger on the knife he was using.

"Tell me where the plasters are," Paul said. "I hate the sight of blood. It makes me faint."

"Then you won't be much help, will you? Go back into the living room, and I will deal with this myself. I'll even make you a cup of coffee."

Paul left the kitchen, and Alex pondered his story. He

suspected Paul was lying. He had smelt alcohol on his breath. After plastering his finger, he continued cooking. He could hear Paul pacing around in the next room, and Alex thought of a caged animal who did not really want to be there. To break the silence he called out, "You can come back in here if you like. I've put a plaster on. The cut wasn't deep."

"It's okay, I'll stay here," Paul called back.

Two hostile animals in a cage are going to fight. The evening had started badly, and Alex knew it was up to him to make it better. He ate his food quickly in the kitchen and then returned to the living room so they could share a bottle of wine. Paul was still pacing and in no mood to talk. Respecting his silence, Alex returned to the kitchen and wondered what the best thing to do was, and at last he decided on his course of action.

"Let's go out and have a drink."

"It's started raining again."

"Never mind about that," Alex said and smiled at Paul. Surprisingly the smile broke the ice.

"I've been a right cunt, haven't I? Keeping you waiting, and then that fuss over blood? I must have sounded a right coward, but it's true I do get faint at the sight of it. That was what I was afraid of this afternoon—that this man would physically hit me. It wouldn't have been the first time."

"Well, you are out of there now. And if you need to give them that money, I am willing to lend it, and let's end the subject there. I've also got an extra raincoat!"

From the wardrobe in the bedroom, he took a long white raincoat. It was another thing he had bought in Paris, but rarely wore. Somehow it worked there, but not in Brighton. He told Paul how the first time he had worn it in Brighton, he had been approached by a woman in Waitrose.

"It's very glamourous," she had said. "Where did you get it?" When he told her he had bought it on the Champs-Élysées, she had laughed and replied, "I saw Charlotte Rampling wearing something similar last year on Eurostar, but it wasn't a patch on yours. I'm sure she would be green with envy."

"You really think so?" he had replied, hoping he was not going to be subjected to any sexual advances.

"By a mile," the woman had replied, and then pushed her trolley away and went off in search of someone else to flirt with.

He handed Paul the raincoat.

"I hope I don't stand out so conspicuously," Paul said, trying the coat on for size. He looked good in it, and as he was taller than Alex, that added to the impression. "I like it," Paul said. "Now, tell me more about Waitrose. I mean, do people actually pick each other up there?"

"It is a bit of a mecca for the solitary. But it's mainly people looking for temporary acquaintances and someone to chat to. I doubt if true romance blossoms there very often."

"I don't think there is a Waitrose in Hull."

Out on the street, the rain was not falling heavily.

"Which pub shall we choose?" Alex asked.

"It's up to you."

"Shall we walk into the centre and find a quiet one?"

In the Lanes, they turned into a side street which had an old-fashioned pub. It was empty, and they took a corner seat.

"The virus keeping them away?" Paul asked.

"Probably," Alex replied and went to get some drinks. He ordered a whisky for himself and a beer for Paul and wondered again how much alcohol Paul had consumed that day. While standing at the bar, his mind decided on an action that might change both of their lives. The flat *was* a cage, and there was no way he was going to move either the bookshelves or the writing desk. He had a plan, possibly a dangerous one, but if Paul was going to become a drunk, it had to be elsewhere.

"Paris," he said as he returned to the table, standing over it with a smile on his face.

"What about it?" Paul asked.

"How would you like to show off your raincoat, walking along the Champs-Élysées?"

"You on something?" Paul joked. "Some substance you haven't told me about?"

"No, I'm not on anything. I couldn't feel clearer than I do now." He sat down, and Paul looked anxiously at him. Then he asked, "Have you got a passport?"

"Yes. It's got a few years left on it."

Alex could feel his own heart beating with excitement as he said, "Then let's go to Paris tomorrow."

"You mean, take a boat?"

"On a rough sea?" Alex joked. "Not on your life. I feel the same way about crossing the Channel as you feel about blood."

"I enjoyed it when I went on a trip to Calais a couple of years ago."

Alex wanted to ask whom he had gone with, or whether he had gone alone, but resisted in case it sounded like an interrogation. He had no intention of prying into Paul's life. What he knew about him was enough.

"We'll go by Eurostar," Alex said.

"Hold on a minute! You just said 'we' as if it was full steam ahead. I've got a job, remember?"

"What is the work exactly? You may have told me, but I've forgotten."

"Nothing much."

"Then leave it and find another when we get back."

"But Alex, you are talking as if I have already agreed."

"Drink your beer and think it over."

Paul gulped down his beer, which left his upper lip smudged with foam. Alex found it sexy, and the acknowledgement of that fact bothered him. The computer is the place for those thoughts, he reminded himself.

"Can I have another beer? I'm wiped out financially. They expect me in tomorrow, and I would have money then—"

"Of course," Alex said, interrupting him and went to get

another drink. He also bought some crisps. He opened the packet, and Paul took one immediately.

"I can't think," Paul said as he munched on it.

"Well then, just accept that we are going."

"This is Rye all over again. I can't *take* from you. It's not what I want to do."

"Pay me back in instalments later."

"Don't be flippant, Alex. How would I be able to do that?" Paul took another crisp and then a further handful. The packet was almost empty before he spoke again. "I like crisps," he said. His voice once again had a childish tone.

"You were hungry," Alex observed.

"So?"

"I did offer you a meal."

"And now you're offering me Paris. What are you, a closet sugar daddy?"

"I'm being honest with you, Paul. I want and I *need* to go to Paris. The flat I normally stay in over there is free at the moment."

"So, you've been planning this?"

Alex felt hostilities were about to take place, and he tried to calm Paul down.

"I was on my way to Paris when we met, remember? I've seen a house less than two hours from Paris, and I should go and see it."

"Oh, that fucking crazy idea of yours!"

"Aren't you even remotely tempted to come with me?" Alex asked.

"To see Paris? Of course I am. It's on my wish list. Who can die without having seen the Mona Lisa? I'm joking about that, I've seen all I need to of her, and I doubt the painting's as great as it's supposed to be. The mysterious smile? What of it? If she has a secret, it's probably very boring."

"I agree with you."

"And it'll cost a bloody fortune."

"Well, the flat is cheap. The owner is an old acquaintance

of mine from thirty years ago. He lets me have it for a token amount, and the fares on Eurostar are normally quite reasonable at this time of year. It won't cost a fortune."

He had lied about the owner being an old acquaintance from thirty years before, but he had stayed at the flat a few times and the elderly man who owned it liked him. He could have gone alone and left Paul to himself, but he wanted to keep his flat in Brighton as it was. He also dreaded the possibility that he could grow too dependent or fond of Paul, but this he dismissed to the back of his mind along with the rest of the junk in his unconscious. He could not countenance affection or any kind of loving, but nor could he deny that as well as the need to preserve the order of his flat, he felt a strange need for Paul's company. Even a character in a Samuel Beckett play needs another, if only to talk at without getting close to. You are weakening, he thought.

"It's just a big step for me," he continued. "I want to live there, but to be honest with you, I am afraid. I'm afraid because for me this choice, wherever I choose, will be the end of the line, and just once, I'd like someone with me who can look at the place as well."

"You mean to approve or disapprove?" Paul's voice was a bit slurred. He had clearly drunk a lot that day, but he was also smiling. He didn't wait for Alex to answer and continued talking. "Did you mean what you said? Will I be able to pay you back gradually what I owe for this trip?"

"If you can, then yes. But Paul, I really won't need the money back," Alex replied.

"I feel a little drunk," Paul said.

"Are you sober enough to know that this journey has no strings attached? I ask nothing more than the pleasure of your company."

"What a nice posh way of expressing it," Paul replied with a note of sarcasm in his voice. "Paris! When I was a child in Hull, it seemed like the end of the world. My dad said he'd been there once, and he used to describe the city in such detail he sounded like a walking guidebook. My mother said he was inventing it all, but I listened. The descriptions he gave of walking by the river at night! He shocked my mother, talking about the couples making love openly underneath the bridges. I wanted to ask him how they did it in the open like that with passers-by and all, but I was only ten or so, and I knew my mother would have slapped me hard."

"Sounds as if you fell in love with the place back then. Will you come with me?"

"Can I have another beer?"

"I'll get you a drink, but no more alcohol. I don't want you hungover tomorrow, and we have some packing to do tonight."

"I haven't unpacked from earlier yet," Paul quipped. He looked at Alex with his glittering, reddish-brown eyes, and murmured, "I will come with you on one condition."

"What's that?"

"I don't want to be homeless when we get back. Promise me you will let me stay in the flat, whatever happens. Give me time enough to find another house and a job."

"I promise."

"And won't the virus be in Paris? More than here? It's a big city."

"I've got masks for our mouths and noses. That will protect us—and lots of hand gel."

"You're having a laugh. Me in a mask? In Paris? How will anyone get to see my ravaged good looks?"

"So, you *are* vain," Alex joked, and reaching over, poked Paul in the chest.

The contradictions that torture the self are obscure. Suddenly Alex regretted asking him. He would be a burden, and he would treat the whole trip as an adventure. He wanted to crawl back into his shell and go to Paris by himself.

"Are you sure about me staying on?" Paul asked.

"Yes. Yes. Yes. Shall I put it on paper or something?"

Alex felt irritated with himself. He wanted to go back in

time to that moment in the bar before he had come up with this idea. So much for impulse! This is the way we play with ourselves.

"Let's go back to the flat," Alex suggested.

Walking in the drizzle, side by side, each of them had their own thoughts. More and more, Alex believed he had let loose a host of demons, and God knows what Paul was thinking. They were silent until they reached the flat and then after a few banal words, Alex shut himself in the toilet, and without a sound, he cried—hard tears, brutal tears that seemed to burn their way down his cheeks. I cannot live with this, he thought over and over again, and he remained in the toilet for at least half an hour, not caring what Paul was thinking or doing. When he came out, Paul looked at him and asked if he was alright. Alex did not answer his question but said that he was giving Paul his bed that night and that he would sleep on the sofa.

"Why?"

"I have some papers to sort out in this room, and you need your sleep."

"So do you."

"Yes, but I can survive on a few hours. I can always sleep on the train to Ashford tomorrow."

"Is that the way we are we going? Through Rye?" Paul asked.

"It's quieter and easier to check in. Would you prefer St. Pancras? We might have to leave earlier."

"I think I would."

"Okay. Agreed. Now, do you agree to sleep in the bedroom?" Paul said he would, and Alex told him he would wake him early so they could have a good breakfast, and that Paul could sleep until he had prepared it. "Now, get as much sleep as you can. Remember you will probably have a bit of a hangover in the morning."

"It's true. I did drink quite a lot today. With the last of my money. Before I came. I was depressed. I didn't want you—to get the wrong impression."

"About what?"

"That I might have a drinking problem. I just get drunk occasionally, that's all."

"Understood," Alex said and gently with his hand he reached out and touched Paul's face. "Your life is your own. And so is mine. We do not have to apologise to each other about anything. We may stand together, but we are alone."

"In a lonely place," Paul whispered. "I get the point."

Paul used the bathroom, had a quick shower, and then closed the bedroom door behind him.

Alex sat on the sofa and waited until there was total quiet. He looked around the room, and after a momentary sigh, began what he had to do. He brought out two suitcases from behind the sofa, and towards four in the morning, he had finished packing everything except for some clothes that were in the bedroom. He set up the sofa-bed and lay there with the light on, drifting in and out of uneasy sleep and bad dreams. In one dream, he was attacked by an infected insect: an insect whose bite had no cure. A doctor with a mask covering his face told him it was hopeless. Alex awoke in a sweat and looked at the clock beside him. It was six in the morning. He shivered in the way people do when they are going down with an illness. He felt his forehead. No temperature.

"I am a fool," he said aloud and then took down a book and read the words in it without following their meaning. His mind was elsewhere in what could only be described as a terrible land.

As the Eurostar sped into the tunnel, Paul gripped Alex by the arm. "Does it go down deep? I'm not sure I'm going to like this."

"I was nervous the first time," Alex answered, "but there is a remedy. Let's go to the bar."

"How far away is it?"

"Two carriages."

"They sell alcohol?"

Alex did not reply to this but stood up and began to walk down the aisle. Paul followed him, and once in the bar, Alex could see that he was immediately more relaxed.

"Can I have some brandy?" Paul asked.

The train seemed to be moving faster than it usually did in the tunnel, and Alex swayed a little as he ordered the drinks. He also got crisps for Paul.

"You do look good in your raincoat," he said, knowing he had to engage in meaningless dialogue to pass the time.

"I felt claustrophobic back there and couldn't wear the mask—with all those people around. It was a risk."

"Just wash your hands or use your hand gel if you touch anything that other people have touched."

"I'm gonna look an awful prat in a mask."

"Pretty soon everyone will be wearing them, believe me. And although it may be over-cautious, I suggest when we arrive at the apartment that we wipe all the surfaces. There probably hasn't been anyone there for a long time, but we might as well."

Then suddenly as if they both needed to relieve the tension, they spontaneously burst out laughing. The mood changed, and Alex saw how happy Paul looked, and it was true, he did look smart in his raincoat. He was also wearing a pair of jeans and had gelled his hair back, which revealed his features and accentuated his *beau-moche* looks. Alex almost envied him.

They came out of the tunnel, and Paul stared at the landscape. He commented on how much space there was in comparison to cramped England, especially in the south-east.

"Yes," Alex breathed deeply. "So much space. I love this country—its size and its shape. It's a hexagon, and it sits solidly and firmly among its neighbours. I like that. I like the shape of France, almost like an attraction to the shape of a person."

Paul did not respond. He was too fixated on what was passing outside the window to answer. He pointed to a distant village with a church spire at its heart. All around, there was countryside, endless countryside, and the sun was shining.

"Is Illiers-Combray like that?"

"I've only seen it on the internet," Alex replied.

"If it looks as pretty as that, it should be a nice place to live, but all the same, it's isolated. Can you bear that kind of isolation?"

"The village you have just seen is practically in the middle of nowhere. Illiers-Combray is close to Chartres, and Paris is a short train journey away. I think in Combray—let's call it that—knowing I was near such great places, I would not feel so isolated."

"All the same," Paul murmured, "supposing they find out you're gay? Villages anywhere are not very gay places."

"I'm not going there to be gay, Paul."

"To use a cliché, Alex, a leopard cannot change its spots. It can't be hidden. Nor should it be. Look, Hull is not an unfriendly place. It has Pride every year, and the occasional gay play or film, but you don't want to be too visible there. D'you know what I mean?"

"Don't you mean *you* don't want to be too visible there?"

"Now we're getting serious, and I don't want to be," Paul said, changing the subject.

"I'll get you another brandy."

"No, just more crisps."

At the bar, Alex spoke in French, and when he returned with the crisps, Paul commented that he would never understand the language. The words flowed too quickly into each other. He added that he had had French lessons at school, but that he only remembered a few words.

"Well, that's a beginning," Alex replied, sipping at the whisky he had ordered for himself.

"How long do you think it would take for me to be able to follow a French film in a cinema?"

"That would depend on the film, but after about nine months, things would start to slot into place. There would be gaps in your comprehension of course, but in time, gaps are filled. It depends on the person, but despite forgetting your schoolboy French, I sense you may be quick to learn."

"Maybe we could start by you pointing out objects to me in French and then me repeating the word after you? It could be a game while we're there. That's if you don't find the idea too boring."

Once more, Alex looked at Paul, and the more he talked with him on the train in this simple and dare he say it happy way, the more relaxed he felt with him. He liked the stranger who would always be Paul. Even so, he had firmly decided that he must not be tempted to get too close to him and that he would encourage Paul to explore Paris by himself. This was for Paul's sake as well as his own. He needed to breathe among the solitude of others and not to have to talk to anyone.

"I'll pick up a copy of Le Monde when we arrive, and then in the flat tonight, you can try to read bits of it aloud, and some of what you learnt at school may come back to you. We can also pick out a few words and discuss their meanings."

"Yes, sir," Paul said mockingly.

Alex got Paul's irony, but did not respond, and simply said, "Shall we go back to our seats?"

"First place I want to see is the Champs-Élysées. But I'll wear my mask. Who knows, it might start a trend. The French can probably make anything fashionable."

"I can see your father told you quite a lot about how Parisians live."

Paul grinned, his wolf eyes creasing up appealingly into narrow slits, and he stared hard at Alex. "I was just thinking," he said. "I don't believe you would want to know who the real me is."

On arrival, fewer masks were being worn than Paul had imagined. "I thought everyone would be wearing them except foolish tourists," he said.

Seen from the taxi, the streets seemed as lively as ever, especially around the Gare du Nord. The taxi driver drove them silently (unusual for a Paris taxi driver) down the main boulevards and then through the narrow streets of the Marais to where they were staying near Saint-Paul.

"Usually they talk more," Alex commented.

At the entrance to the building, Alex buzzed open the heavy front door with the code the owner, Claude, had emailed him. Inside, they faced a steep flight of stairs. "We're up on the second floor," he said.

Claude had left the key to the apartment in a concealed panel on the second-floor landing. When they entered and turned on the lights, they were confronted by a vase filled with flowers. It was Claude's way of saying "Welcome."

After they put their luggage down, Alex wiped his hands with gel and suggested they start immediately to clean the surfaces in the apartment. Paul remarked that surely Claude had cleaned the place before their arrival, but Alex replied it was a good habit for them both to get into.

It was immediately clear to Paul why the owner only let the place out to a select few. It was a small but beautiful apartment. The walls were covered with original paintings which Alex explained were by some fairly well-known artists, bought back in the 1960s when Claude was young. Apparently, he was wealthy and had inherited the house he lived in from his parents. The apartment itself had been acquired to give extra space for his guests, back when the Marais was still run-down and unfashionable. Alex had been introduced to Claude as a writer and that had appealed to him, and since then, although they had never become close, Alex had always found the apartment was available to him, even at short notice. He charged little, operating no doubt on the assumption that to charge the high prices others did was a vulgarity he would not sink to, and Alex sensed that Claude was now essentially solitary like himself.

Paul hadn't lost his enthusiasm for seeing the Champs-Élysées on their first evening, but after cleaning the apartment, buying essential food at the local supermarket, and eating a simple meal in a bistro on the corner, it was clear they were both exhausted.

"We'll go tomorrow," Alex said to a visibly disappointed Paul.

"Who gets to sleep on the sofa?" Paul asked.

"You take the bed in the other room."

"But that's not fair."

"The sofa makes a good bed. I assure you I will be comfortable."

After Paul closed the bedroom door, Alex sat on the sofa and surveyed the room. He looked at the objects in the room, paying close attention to each of the paintings and the sketches. Then he looked at the furniture: at the chairs and the table which were made of grey iron. They were idiosyncratic but aesthetic. In contrast, there was an old wooden chest of drawers: a rustic piece of furniture that showed its age well. The object filled him with an uneasy peace. Once more, Alex had a sleepless night.

The next day did not begin well. It started with glances, as if an unspoken hatred between them was coming to the surface, and in those glances was wariness: a fear of hatred and of another unspoken emotion that could not be named but which existed somewhere between longing and repulsion.

Paul paced the room impatiently, staring at the paintings, looking at them with anger as if they were too rich for his taste and that he was inferior to them.

Alex feared Paul's strength and also his weakness. He

feared that Paul could tear him apart, but that first, his wolf eyes would enchant him into a realm of emotion he did not want to enter.

"I want to go out," Paul said. "You said you would show me Paris. Show me Paris."

It was an order and not a request, and in the heat of the moment, Alex replied, "For God's sake, just take a map and some money. Go and explore by yourself and leave me alone to do what I have to do."

"No! I don't want that. I've come with you, and I'm going to stay with you until I've seen the whole city. What about the French you were going to teach me from the newspaper? What about all the stuff I can only learn from you? I'm not some street boy you've just picked up, to be thrown back onto the streets because you're bored. I will *not* be alone."

"I need my solitude," Alex said.

"You said before you needed my companionship, that you needed someone with you. Why are you contradicting yourself?"

"I'm sorry, perhaps it would be better if you returned to England."

"I just want to see new things. I want to see the Eiffel Tower. I want to see the Moulin Rouge, and don't you have to rediscover Paris, as you want to live so near it and visit so often? Or are you at last seeing sense and realising that you cannot achieve your goal? Is that why you're so miserable?"

"Stop it, Paul. I have to act before it is too late."

"Too late for what?"

"Before I become too old to act, and before the drawbridge is taken up on both sides of the channel. I'm not rich enough to pay for private healthcare or to do without the state pension in the future. There's only a narrow window of time left in this transition year: the last few months for me to achieve stability." He paused, then shouted, "For fuck's sake, don't you understand?"

"No, I don't. Not this panic in you. If you have to stay in

your country, England—"

"It's not my country."

"Your country. You may have to stay. Accept."

"I can't."

"You can't accept anything, really can you? I see it in your eyes: a fear that despises; that despises even me because I am too English for you. Why don't you admit it? It has come to the surface here, hasn't it? The divide between us? That you want to be French and that I am your enemy, the Englishman."

"There is another virus that is separating us, and that is hate."

"Did I say I felt any hate, any dislike towards you?"

Alex went into the kitchen and like a robot, went about the business of preparing food. There was silence in the living room. Thinking that everything was calm, Alex returned into the room and said, "There are eggs, ham, and bread. I'm hungry. You must be hungry. We have to eat."

"Sod the bloody food," Paul cried out, and as Alex turned his back on him, he heard a crash. Paul had ripped a picture from the wall and thrown it to the floor. The glass was smashed.

"You little bastard," Alex said, rushing at Paul. He grabbed him by the throat and pushed him against the wall. Violence and hatred flowed between them like an electric current. Paul fought back and kicked out his legs with rapid and persistent force. He kicked Alex's legs several times, and then in the groin. Alex released his grasp. Paul rushed at his throat and shouted, "I gonna fucking kill you."

Alex fought him off and cried out, "Don't you realise what you've done? How this will upset Claude? A man you don't even know. The glass is broken and the frame. It's a very old frame. Irreplaceable. You really are a bastard," Alex repeated and flopped down onto the sofa. Paul came over, rubbing at his throat and looked down at him.

"Give me the map of Paris," he said coldly, "and the

money. I'll be out all day. I suppose you will let me in again?"

"You have the code. Just come up the stairs and ring the bell."

"Weren't there two sets of keys? Can't I let myself in?"

Alex was in shock at what had happened. He got up, picked up a set of keys, and in silence he handed them to Paul. He then took a map of Paris and gave it to him. "Here," he said, holding it out.

"And how am I supposed to get around?"

"However you want. Walk. Take the Metro. There's a Metro plan on the map. Ask for a *carnet* of ten tickets. And here," he said, handing out a wad of Euro notes, "this will be more than enough for whatever you want to do."

Paul took the notes without checking how much was there and put them in his pocket. "We have to get over this," he said, his voice quiet. He too seemed shocked at their row and at what he had done.

Alex could not answer. Just looking at Paul made him feel sick. He saw the mark on Paul's neck that he had made, but he did not care. His groin hurt him badly. "I've got a lot of calls to make. It will take me all day. I have arrangements to make. Come back as late as you like."

"Don't worry, I will make this day last as long as I can." Paul then went to the door, and as he reached for the latch, he burst into tears. "I was happy on the train," he said, wiping his eyes. "What happened? What *is* happening between us? You can't stand the sight of me. Coming here has stripped us of our friendship, of everything."

"Perhaps it has brought our very different sufferings to the surface."

"Yes, perhaps," Paul replied.

Alex continued by saying, "What is causing yours, I cannot and do not want to know. As for mine, I can express it in one word, one name. Luc. He was the one man I truly loved, and although it's long ago, I cannot accept the pain I caused him. Everything in this city reminds me of him."

"I hope he's dead!" Paul said savagely as he left, slamming the door behind him.

Left alone, Alex was both relieved and exhausted. Paul's last terrible words echoed in his head, and his mind was so full that he thought he would go mad. All past conversations with Paul had left his memory or had sifted down into the darkest part of his inner self. What had he told him about Luc? Had he in fact said *anything* about him? He paced the room and then to do something that would distract him, he put the smashed picture in a bag, and went out. After making a few enquiries, he found a shop in the area that could repair it within a couple of days. Returning to the apartment, the mark on the wall where it had been became a dismal focal point, almost an accusation. His instinct told him to contact Claude and tell him, but he did not have the courage. It was not that he was afraid Claude might tell him to leave, he simply did not want to hurt the man with his admission. He hoped the repair shop would do a good job and that Claude would not notice at all. The violence within him returned, and he wanted to hit Paul repeatedly. This thought disturbed him so much that he went into the bedroom where Paul had slept, and looking down at the crumpled sheets, fell to his knees, buried his face in them, and cried. He could smell the odour of Paul's body, and perversely the smell excited him and yet repelled him. He got to his feet and went back into the living room. He distracted himself for the next hour by trying to reach the agent for the house, and when finally he got through, he announced in a gush that he had the money and wanted to buy the house. At first, the agent was silent, perhaps surprised by his English accent and the urgency in his voice, but after Alex explained his situation further, the agent informed him that the house had been on the market for a long while and that the price had recently been reduced by a several thousand Euros. He more or less assured Alex that the owner would accept any serious offer, especially as Alex was a cash buyer, but then came the shock. It would not be possible to visit the house for four weeks, due to a lack of keys and the unavailability of the owner. Nevertheless, an appointment was agreed in four weeks' time, and the conversation ended. "It has to happen," Alex repeated to himself like a mantra, and listening to his own positive words, the heaviness in his head lifted, and he felt a tentative peace. He had taken action. Returning to the bedroom, he undressed, got into bed and slept.

When he awoke, he was shocked to find Paul in bed beside him. He was not sleeping but looking at him. His right hand reached out and touched Alex's stomach.

"Don't," Alex said, but at the same time, he felt he had to let go, to give in. Paul moved closer, and after a light kiss on Alex's lips, he moved his head downwards to suck on one of Alex's nipples. Then he began kissing Alex's stomach, and at the same time fondled his penis. Nothing in Alex wanted this to happen, but in the mental country of contradictions he was in, he knew that he would let it happen; that it had to happen. Paul was not gentle with him, and his penetration was painful. After the act, they lay side by side in bed, and Paul said, "I'm sorry for everything."

"Are you sorry about this?" Alex asked.

"No. I wanted it. I knew I had to make amends for the way I behaved."

His words were strangely ambiguous, and Alex said, "It sounds as if you offered yourself to make up for something; that you would not have done this if this morning hadn't happened."

"No, it's not like that."

"Then how is it, Paul?"

"Please don't question. It was bad for me out there, alone in the streets. I didn't get the Metro. I walked. First, I walked in a straight line to a square which had a couple of theatres."

"Châtelet," Alex said.

"Yeah. I remember the name. Then I cut down to the Seine,

and despite how awful I felt, I liked the view across the river, but it was only liking. There was no real attraction. I couldn't love this city the way you do. I saw a few people with masks on, and the fear hit me that I had left mine here. I'd have liked to go into a café, but I didn't want to touch the surfaces, 'cos I left the hand gel here as well."

"I'll take you somewhere you'll like later."

"Will that mean taking the Metro and being crowded together?"

The voice of the child; a very young child who is terrified of pain and the possibility of illness. Alex remembered his own voice long ago when he'd had influenza, and nothing could take away the fear. Even at the age of eight, he saw death as a final darkness and a void. His mother had not comforted him, and no one told him not to be afraid. Paul had the same desolate voice.

"We'll go by taxi and see the city by night, safely."

Paul got out of the bed and went to the bathroom to take a shower. Alex listened to the splashing of the water, and his repulsion and hatred towards Paul went away. Hate is like a long stairway downwards to the night of the soul, and Alex knew that fortunately he had only descended one step. He got out of bed and put on his clothes. When he went into the living room, he found Paul staring at the empty space where the picture had been.

"Where is it now?" he asked with his back to Alex.

"I took it to be repaired. It will be fine. I don't think Claude will ever know."

"But *I* know," Paul replied.

"We must forget. In a couple of days, it will be back in its place."

Paul turned and took Alex in his arms. He hugged him tightly, and all Alex could say was, "It's not important. It really isn't."

"I am violent," Paul whispered and then broke away and added coldly, "But aren't all men?"

About an hour later, they went out.

"It has my name," Paul said, looking up at the church that gave the area of Saint-Paul its name. "It's ugly."

Nearby, there was a restaurant with no name and Alex proposed a meal. They sat on its heated terrace because Paul was nervous about sitting inside and ordered steak and fried potatoes. A table wine was brought to them, and Paul asked if it was any good.

"I used to know the best of wines," Alex replied, "but like a lot of things, I have forgotten the names."

As Alex poured the wine, Paul asked, "Will you remember my name?"

Alex glanced at him and saw another kind of fear on his face: the look of one who is fearful they will never be remembered by anyone.

"You must not have such thoughts," Alex said, sipping at the wine.

The solitary waiter stood nearby, watching them closely. The restaurant was practically empty, and he clearly had nothing else better to do.

"I want to ask you something, Alex. It was while I was out by myself that the thought came to me. I know you will refuse after what happened, and that we are perhaps incompatible, but—"

There was a long silence, and Alex put his knife and fork down. "Go on," he said.

"About us. Companionship. Not love maybe, but not being alone. Being alone for me is worse than the virus." He laughed, and once again, the face creased, but there was no real laughter there. "I know you will say no, so I'd better shut up and forget it."

"No, go on."

"Well, first, about this morning. We didn't really dislike, hate, call it what you like—did we?"

"I think we did, Paul."

"But it wasn't real. It was like a nightmare that continues after you are awake. I was not myself, and I made you not yourself."

"I know I hated myself for hating."

"Then we must never feel that again."

There was a long pause, and then Alex asked, "Can we return to the subject of what you want to ask me?"

Paul finished his glass of wine in one gulp and then stared hard at Alex; the lines in his face hinting at the future that old age would make of it. Alex saw how it would harden if he was not careful. He knew that Paul would age badly and that even his eyes would lose their ginger highlights and become cold and lifeless, and he knew very well that when the light goes out of the eyes, what is revealed is interior death. It is the same for all of us who are solitary, he thought. We fade quietly, and we walk like crippled beings.

"I would like to help you do up this house you want to live in. I have nothing in England. I just want the doing of it, and to know that you won't be unhappy if I am there."

"But you have no relationship with this country."

Paul poured himself the final glass of wine from the carafe.

"Things change. I will change. Things grow," he said."

"But not love—" Alex replied.

"That too could change. I looked at the Seine this afternoon. It was sweeping by so quickly. I thought of time, of how much time we have and too often waste. I thought of all the suicides who have died in the waters, afraid that it was too late to live."

"I can't say yes to this," Alex said.

"Is that final?"

Suddenly, with terrifying ferocity, Alex thought, if you let this request from Paul go, you will regret it. The memory of this dinner in this almost empty restaurant will haunt you like a purgatory, and like those suicides in the river, you might as well jump.

"Look what happened to us earlier," Alex said, "violence, and then that burst of sexuality. Is that how you see us if we carry on together? If you don't see it like that, and sincerely don't see it like that, then yes, you can take your place in the house."

Paul looked at Alex quickly, and the spark of his eyes had the piercing beauty of expectation: the quick flash of light, green, like the green ray that flashes at the moment of sunset before it disappears into the sea. He knew that few ever see that magical sight, but he saw it in Paul's eyes, and he was overwhelmed that Paul had revealed it to him. He was so overwhelmed that he had to get up and go downstairs to the washroom. He had to wash his face with cold water because he felt it was burning. And yet, the contradictions within him remained. Part of him hoped that Paul would no longer be there when he got back to the table, but the other part of him, said no, I do not love him, but dare I need him? Do I feel that? Has it brought me to life again emotionally, that light from his eyes? He washed his face at the sink and gazed at his own face in the mirror. Was there a light too in his eyes, not the same as in Paul's but equally intense? He looked for a confirmation, and he saw it. His eyes were young; as young as when he had been with Luc. He recalled another mirror back in 1986, and vividly his unconscious brought to the surface, the young man he was who had known all too briefly happiness. He raised his hands to his face and saw the fingers that had grasped Paul's throat. In shame he dropped them and looking again in the mirror he still saw the youth he had been. Something told him that there had been no hatred between them, only a cruelty born of frustration. Go forward, his eyes said.

Paul was sitting at the table, looking down at his empty plate.

"Paul, we can try," Alex said.

"No, we can't. You shouldn't have left me alone. I began to think. I had time to think. I would be violent again. I am aware of that within me. Rage. Sudden rage. You don't know all the things I've done in the past."

"I don't need to know."

"Can we pay for the meal?" Paul asked briskly. "Or rather, can *you* pay for the meal? You have no idea how much I still dislike taking money from you." Then he laughed. "But wait! I've forgotten. I can pay, can't I? The money you gave me earlier. I didn't spend a single Euro. At least I will have the appearance of being able to pay. The waiter might even respect me. I'm sure he dislikes us. Thinks we are a couple of queers. His arrogant bored face says that loud and clear, but he might slightly respect the younger of us being the one to cough up the money. I need a modicum of respect, even from him."

"Paul, don't change!" Alex said.

"From what?"

"From the man I left at the table."

"I shouldn't have asked to help you renovate. I'm shit at it anyway. Now I'm going to march up to that arrogant sod and pay, like one male whore who isn't so much of a whore after all."

Alex let him go. He did not watch. The moment has gone, he thought. The green ray had heralded only darkness.

They did not go on to see Paris by night from a taxi. Alex mentioned it, but Paul refused. He was withdrawn and sulky; hollowed out, and his eyes reflected the emptiness inside him. Had Alex's departure for the washroom killed him?

"Can we watch television?" Paul asked when they got back to the apartment.

"It's all in French."

"So?" Paul's voice was aggressive.

"The programmes aren't up to much."

"You mean worse than in England? Isn't it all crime, period dramas and reality shows like it is back there? There must be something worth watching."

Alex walked over to the black rectangle in the corner

which he had so far avoided and turned it on. It was a news programme reporting protests against Roman Polanski being awarded the Best Director *César*. He looked at Paul, who was trying to work out what was going on.

"It's about—" Alex began.

"I know what it's about," Paul interjected. "I've seen some of Polanski's films. I like them. Now they're throwing him to the wolves, aren't they? Look, there's a running line of breaking news beneath the image. I can just about manage to put some of it together."

"Shall I keep it on?"

"Okay by me."

"Do you want some ice cream while we watch?" Alex asked.

"Fine. Yes."

The images on the screen flashed into Paul's face with brittle artificiality. A woman was talking about her abuse, and how Polanski was the perpetrator, and although Alex was dubious about Polanski's offences, he was, along with Paul, someone who appreciated his films. It sounded like a verbal lynching, and he did not like lynchings. He cut himself on a sharp knife he had stupidly tried to use to force the lid of the ice cream open.

"Damn you," he said aloud.

"Nice!" Paul said.

"I mean this knife. I don't want to bleed into the ice cream."

Going back into the room, he saw that the news report had changed to an item on fashion, and a woman was parading down a catwalk in a long coat.

"Doesn't *that* objectify women?" asked Paul. "Why don't they go to fashion shows and shout at them? Anyway, after this, they're showing some comedy about a marriage on the rocks. Shall we watch something on the internet instead?"

Alex turned off the television and Paul asked if he had downloaded anything interesting recently. "A gay film," he added. "Let's have a look in the funny mirror. Gay life in gay films always amuses me. All those straight hunks hiding their pricks whenever they get out of bed or have showers."

"I'll see what I've got," Alex replied. "First of all, I'd better go back and clean up the mess in the kitchen."

When Alex returned into the living room, Paul said, "I've changed my mind. Let's look at BritLads on PornHub."

"Stop it, Paul," Alex answered. He felt dangerously close to descending another step towards hatred.

"Stop what? At least they *look* as if they are enjoying it."

"But why? Why porn?"

"I can come twice in a day. We can wank together," he replied flippantly.

"No way," Alex said and slammed the laptop shut.

Silently, Paul got up and disappeared into the bathroom. When he came out, his hair was gelled down, and he was wearing tight jeans and a broken-down leather jacket that Alex had not seen before.

"Don't wait up for me," Paul said. "I'll sleep on the sofa tonight." He then went to the door and slipped once again out of Alex's life.

The torture screws of little cruelties twisted hard inside Alex. He stayed awake until three in the morning, but there was no sign of Paul. He lay there with his clothes on, and when he eventually fell asleep, he had to fight off the chimaeras that haunted him. Luc appeared in one dream with his face blown off. His mind's unravelling of horrible images seemed endless. Torn from his ragged sleep by the sound of steps and the opening of a door, he awoke, and expected to see Paul in the room, but he was not there, and he realised he had dreamt the sounds.

The day eventually dawned, and he ate a couple of French toasts for breakfast but was not hungry enough to eat more. In the cold light of the morning, he sat on the floor and wondered how long he should wait. Drained of feeling, he listened to the various noises in the house. A radio was playing upstairs, and below in the street, he heard the occasional honking of car horns and scooters. He leant his head out of the window. An old car was parked below; it was green, from an era long ago, and an elderly man was sitting in it. A woman from the next house came out and got into it, and they drove away. This sight triggered memories of even older cars coming down to Brighton from London each November and finishing their drive on Marine Parade. Would he miss Brighton, he wondered and decided that yes, he would, but that he would get over it. He reviewed in his mind all the places of so-called beauty in the city, but there was no warmth inside of him as the images came to mind. He recalled how the front and especially the back of the Royal Pavilion looked as if they desperately needed a new coat of paint. He saw the building sites and scaffolding in Kemp Town, at the hospital and other places, their ugliness adding to the city's pockmarked disarray. "One day they might get it right," he said aloud, and then shook his head. He knew they would fail, and that the greed to build and the laziness to renew old buildings would be just the same as before. Not once during these thoughts did he think of Paul, but when he looked at his watch and saw it was midday, he decided to go out.

This was Paris by himself and for himself. The streets in the fourth arrondissement were not crowded, and he walked to the Bastille where he found a café and sat for a full hour watching the people passing. A few were wearing masks, but no more than on the previous days. Leaving the table for a moment, he crossed to the news kiosk that was facing him and bought Le Monde. He read a few articles about the virus, and a piece on Polanski, but he learnt nothing he did not already know and put the paper aside. He drank his coffee and nibbled on a croissant. The sky was overcast, but there was no rain. He paid the waiter who had been flirting with a pretty young woman seated at the back of the terrace. He looked irritated that Alex was waiting for his change. Alex smiled at the young woman, but she looked through him with an empty gaze. Clearly, he did not interest her in any way. Probably she could see that he was too old. Defiant, he decided to find out if he was too old for gay men, and retraced his steps back to Saint-Paul and into the Marais. He passed Les Mots à la Bouche, and saw a sign warning of their impending closure, but he did not go in to find out more. Books were meaningless to him at present, and with a certain cynicism, he told himself that he had read most of what was essential and that the rest was ephemera. Books could involve, but they were not life, and he pondered the possibility that he might never write again. What more was there to say? The stories of this new age were in the future, and the past was well and truly in the past. 2020 was a point of renewal, but with the threat of an impending pandemic, he had a pessimistic vision of how society would be changed. 2020 like 1920 would mark the true beginning of the new century. The first twenty years had been nothing more than growing pains, but that had all ended on December 31st. He told himself that with luck (or was it?) he would survive a few more decades and then? Nothing. A no more; as if by being pushed out of life, he would be pushed into oblivion, and oblivion meant never knowing he had existed or what it had felt like. This sombre realisation denied an afterlife, and it was while he was still contemplating these questions that he entered the Café Cox and ordered a whisky.

"Alexander?"

At first, he did not believe it was a call to him, but when his name was repeated, he turned and saw, sitting at a table, a man much older than him. Hesitantly he went over, and looking down at the white hair, the pale face and shrunken figure, he had no recall and no idea whom the man might be.

"You don't remember me?" the man asked.

"I'm sorry, but no, I don't."

"We knew each other in 1985. Only for a few days—a good few days. I introduced you to Pierre Boulez and to his music. You neither liked it nor tried to understand it, but I was patient with you. I am Sylvain."

Intrigued by this figure of the past of whom he had no recollection whatsoever, he sat down with his drink and faced him.

"I remember you were afraid of human contact back then. Are you still?"

"I must apologise," responded Alex, "but I really do not recall our meeting. I rarely went out onto the scene then."

"Yes, you told me that. You were teaching, weren't you? Teaching the young how to speak English?"

"Yes, that is correct," Alex replied.

"Your French accent is still very good, as it was then. I had an apartment in Saint-Cloud. I took you there, and we spent two days together. Then you got afraid, or so it seemed to me. We made no promises to meet again, and I felt a great sadness when you left."

The word sadness, *tristesse*, hung in the air between them—a lost memory like the forgetting of a poem by Verlaine. A voice inside him said that it had to be Verlaine: the poet of tristesse.

"There's a poem that has come into my mind by Verlaine. I don't know why. I cannot quite bring the words forward."

Sylvain smiled, but Alex had difficulty seeing his eyes properly because he was wearing dark glasses. It was clear that he did not want to take them off.

"Perhaps it is *Dernier espoir*?" Sylvain suggested. "Maybe you can recall the last three lines:

Ah, vivre encor ! Mais quoi, ma belle,
Le néant est mon froid vainqueur...
Du moins, dis, je vis dans ton coeur ?"

Sylvain's voice trembled as he recited this softly, and bending forward, Alex asked, "Did you really read that poem to me? Back then?"

"Yes. I gave you the Pléiade edition of Verlaine's *Oeuvres poétiques complètes*."

Alex felt a pain inside. It hit hard in his chest. This man, this man whose name was Sylvain, was buried, buried deep. The pain reminded him yet again that memory failed, and that it invented as well, and that each person has separate souvenirs.

"I was a stranger to you then, and I am a stranger now. Isn't that the truth, Alexander?"

"Yes, and the poem, for me, seems never to have been recited or read by either of us before."

Sylvain raised a cup to his lips and asked how Alex was after all those years. Alex told him he was intending to move back to France.

"Is that wise?"

"I think so."

"To Paris?"

"No, Sylvain. Illiers-Combray. I've seen a house there. It needs a certain amount of renovation, but I like it. It has one room in particular that appeals to me."

"Can you describe it?"

"I've only seen a photo of it, but I will try. There is a fireplace of brown stone, framed as if it were a picture—a square picture with a wooden surround—and this impression is accentuated by the brown flagstones on the floor. On either side of the fireplace are tall white antique cupboards set into the wall. Nothing jars and they intrude in no way at all. Above, there are brown wooden beams spanning the whole of the ceiling, and there are two tall windows which let in the light. Fine white curtains flutter inwards as both windows are open."

"A quiet room for a quiet man," Sylvain said. "How old are you now, Alexander?"

"Approaching sixty."

"And I am approaching eighty. When we met, our age difference interfered, I think. I think you were looking for someone younger. Did you find him? Did you love him?"

"Please, Sylvain, I do not want to go back to that time. Yes, I did meet someone. It was 1986. A terrible year. I beg you not to ask any more."

"Of course not. I hope I have not embarrassed you by calling you over. My sight is failing, but something in the way you moved made me think that it was you."

Alex then asked politely if he could get Sylvain another drink.

"No, one is enough. I live in a small apartment nearby. I come here sometimes, just to remind myself that life continues, but often I do not go out at all, and as I cannot read much, the hours pass slowly. It is good at this time of day to hear the sound of voices."

Sadness still hung between them, and Alex had to ask, "Why do you remember me? What was so special back then?"

"I thought you did not want to talk about it, but I will go on, just a little. Those two days we had were enough for me to fall in love with you. I took a photo of you. I still have it in the apartment. You look evasive, as if you wanted to get away. But you affected me, Alexander, in a way that no one else has." He paused, and then added, "I never told you that I loved you, and the reason why is even clearer to me now than it was back then. You were not really aware of my existence. Now that I know you have completely forgotten me, I too will try to forget. I have few years left, and I want to depart this life without any emotional lingering. There is nothing worse in the ordeal of dying than the intrusion of lost love. Love itself is the most important thing in life, and I do not want to recall what I failed to achieve; a reciprocal response."

"Sylvain, I—"

"No. Now you must quietly go. There is nothing left. The fire is out."

"I will remember this encounter—if that means anything."

Sylvain raised his head. It was a noble head, a proud head, and he took off his glasses. His faded blue eyes were looking at him, but Alex noticed that they seemed to drift to one side, towards the distant bar. Sylvain replaced his glasses and smiled. "You are still handsome," he said.

Alex stood up. He felt he should either shake hands or kiss Sylvain on the cheek, but he could do neither. He did not have the right. Why could he not remember those lost two days?

"Take care," Sylvain said.

"You too," Alex said, and whispering a soft goodbye, he left the Café Cox.

After buying some groceries, he went back to the apartment, no longer caring whether Paul had returned or not. He turned on the television, but it was a discussion about the Coronavirus, and he turned it off. He recalled the long night in Brighton he had spent trying to recall the years he had spent in Paris in the 1980s, but Sylvain was not there, and even now after seeing him it was as if he had never been there. To be loved, and not to know it. He took a long shower and had one single desire: to make himself clean. Once dressed, he had a spartan meal of mixed salad, tuna and a glass of wine. The hours went by, and he counted the days until his appointment with the estate agent in Illiers-Combray. He opened the second of his suitcases, which he had not opened since his arrival, and took out a book. It was a battered copy of André Gide's diaries, and he started to read. He read for a couple of hours and then put the book down. He realised that the thought of Paul opening the door and coming back in horrified him.

"I must go out again," he said to himself.

He walked further this time. Through various side streets, he reached the Seine and looked towards the wounded form of Notre-Dame. He did not wish to approach it. His goal was to cross the river, to walk along the Boulevard Saint-Germain, and to have a last drink in the Café de Flore: the former meeting place of so many homosexuals. He doubted there would be any now. He knew what Grindr had done to destroy those waitings, those anticipations of desire, those hopes of sitting beside a desirable stranger, and the extended foreplay of mutual attention that would be played out like a silent Marivaux play. Did such silent theatre still exist between men? Were there some who still preferred the playing, the expectation of the game, whether for sex or eventual loving? It was a question he could not answer, but he hoped that foolish romanticism still existed. A non-believer can still believe in the beauty of the ritual. As he passed the Sainte-Chapelle, he decided to turn back, and when he reached Châtelet, he took the Metro to the Champs-Élysées. He thought of Paul, and the intensity of that thought, urged him to make the journey he had promised him on that first day. He got out at Franklin D. Roosevelt and found there were not so many people on the Avenue. Again, some were wearing masks, and for the first time he sensed that strangers, wary of each other, were keeping their distance. His mind drifted to *Le Grand Meaulnes* and the masks worn at the ball in the lost *manoir* in the heart of Sologne, to the dancing and excitement that a masked face can bring, but none of that existed now. The mask was now a symbol of fear, of dread and of self-preservation. Could it be that the long festival, the long years of the party were coming to an end?

"Paul, where are you?" he murmured as he looked around him. "Why don't you surprise me as Sylvain did? Have you forgotten me as I had forgotten him?"

He walked down the escalator into the FNAC and found the shop almost empty. He wanted to buy a DVD to watch when he returned to the apartment. His eyes scanned the covers, and in the drama section *Sauvage* caught his eye. He read the blurb and decided to get it. He remembered having been impressed by the lead actor Félix Maritaud in another film but could not recall the title. He noticed that people were standing warily apart from each other as they queued to pay, and when it was his turn, he suddenly realised he had not brought out any hand gel to clean his hands afterwards. He felt a moment of panic: his first true panic concerning the invisible threat, and hurrying back into the street, he made his way to the nearest café. Paranoia begins now, he thought to himself, and instead of ordering a drink, he rushed down the stairs and headed towards the toilet, the water and the soap. He left the café immediately afterwards, and instead of taking the Metro decided, tired though he was, to walk back to Saint-Paul. He was afraid of other people.

As he walked up the stairs to the apartment, he could hear the sound of the television. Paul had returned. He opened the door, and found Paul seated on the floor, watching a gameshow. Without saying anything, Alex went to the bedroom and noticed that one of his suitcases had been tampered with. In the kitchen, he made some coffee, and glancing into the main room, he saw that Paul was in the same position, but he also noticed how tense his body was. He asked Paul whether he would like to share the coffee with him.

"No." The reply was terse, angry.

Returning to the kitchen, Alex drank his coffee alone, and afterwards he ran a bath. He locked the door and watched the water flow into the tub. He wanted Paul to leave. He wanted to sink into the water, to be cleansed, and then to return into the room and find him gone, but he had to wait as he had forgotten to add any cold water and the bath was far too hot. He stood facing the mirror. It was hazed over, and he wiped it clean with his hands. He looked at himself, and an old man stared back at him; the old man he would eventually become. His hair seemed greyer. His skin was taut, and deep dark rings surrounded his eyes. In the hollows that contained his vision, a frightened look stared back. He jolted backwards and almost fell into the bath. He was suddenly afraid of taking off his clothes; afraid he would see the fragility of his body in the same way he had seen his face. He sat on the rim of the bath, still clothed, then pulling the plug, he let the water drain away.

There was a knock on the door, and he did not respond. A second knock, and Paul's loud voice said, "I need to piss. Will you be long?"

Alex opened the door and pushed by Paul's waiting figure. He went into the main room, turned off the television, and could hear the sound of Paul urinating. The sound seemed louder than anything that had come from the inane game show, and he felt revulsion. He heard the flush and Paul's heavy tread as he came back into the main room.

"Don't ask me where I've been," Paul said loudly.

Alex said nothing. He had his back to him.

"Well, don't you want to hear?"

"Oh, just shut up," Alex replied.

"I fucked a good little Paris boy. Barely spoke a word of English. He liked my cock. He said he liked English porn and that he thought English cocks were the best. He said the veins showed more and he liked pronounced veins on a hard cock."

"He barely spoke English, and he managed to say all that?" Alex responded slowly, his back still turned to Paul. He felt vulnerable as he had no idea what Paul was capable of. Did he have a knife from the kitchen? The sharp one for cutting meat? He imagined Paul plunging it into his back and expected it would feel like cold ice. The prospect of this cold thrust scared him, and yet at the same time, he thought, let it happen.

"When I said barely, I meant he could understand most things, but expressed himself badly in return. He said he would like to love me, and I laughed in his face. Shall I show you how I laughed in his face?"

Alex heard the taunting voice, and knew there would be no knife, but there could be violence. To avoid it or to face it, he decided to turn around, and he stared at Paul's face. "Go on," he said. "Do it. Do whatever your twisted mind wants to do. I know your anger is about to explode."

"Why don't you hit me?" Paul cried out.

Alex smiled. "Why should I?" Alex said. "To bring the violence out into the open? I have no idea why we should fight as I really do not care about this boy, what you did with him or where you did it. I want to make that quite clear. Any violence you have in you towards me, I give you permission to express. Personally, I have nothing to give you. Not even my fists."

Paul stepped back like a defeated child. An old child. He looked older than Alex had looked in the bathroom mirror.

"Question me, for God's sake," Paul said.

"I told you, I don't care. You called him a boy. Was he underage? Is that what you really like? In Paris, you see, there is a sort of tradition—not politically correct at the moment—of going with fourteen, fifteen-year-olds. Seventeen at the max. They call them *minets*, which if memory serves me correctly, means kittens. At least that is how I translated it when I lived here. Once past eighteen, a boy becomes a man and is no longer a *minet*." He paused, glad that Paul was quiet, and glad too that he was no longer a physical threat. And yet, just as he had desired to feel the ice-cut of the knife, he still regretted it was not yet all over for him. The life that appeared before him seemed no longer worth living.

"He was twenty," Paul said.

"*Le bel âge!*" Alex replied, and brushing past Paul, returned to the kitchen. He needed a glass of water. Paul followed him in.

"I thought you'd suffer because I had disappeared," he said.

"Did you? Well, you will never know. But to be practical for a moment, can I ask you why you went through my suitcase?" He then took Paul by the arm and led him into the bedroom. Paul stared down at the dishevelled contents.

"I don't know."

"Of course you do."

"No, I just wanted to see what was in it. I had no reason. I apologise."

Alex sat on the bed and put his head in his hands. "Do you mind sleeping on the sofa, Paul. I'm exhausted, and I need this bed tonight."

"Sure." Paul left the room and closed the door behind him.

Alex lay on the bed, fully clothed, with the lights on, and stared up at the ceiling which was pealing slightly in the corners. An end had been reached, but he knew that beyond all the anger and the violence, Paul was hurting, and he did not want him to feel pain. His emotions were not so enquiring as to want to learn more or go deeper into Paul's motivations and desires. He just wanted the cleanness of a break, but it had to be done carefully, and anyway, he was still his temporary responsibility. He had brought him to France; an act that in itself implied feeling, even if most of it was now lost. Then in his mind, he saw Sylvain's face. He saw the dark glasses and heard a voice that had spoken to him years before, and that he had forgotten. He wanted suddenly to leave the apartment and to try to find him again. Soon Sylvain would be the last piece of the jigsaw puzzle of his past, and selfishly he wanted to be seen by eyes that had known him and that still knew him. Sylvain, the stranger who had been in love with him, was it he who would be the final representation of so many years gone by? His urge to re-find him was intense. "One last mirror," he said to himself quietly. "One last mirror in which to gaze at all the foolishness and errors and lack of loving." He stood up as if to go out. But what would a man so old be doing out so late? He fantasised that Sylvain might perhaps be unable to sleep and that he would take a walk around the Marais. He fantasised that they would meet, and that he, Alex, would take the old man by the hand and sit with him on a bench, and that despite the cold outside, the warmth of their encounter would banish the weather and anything else that could separate them. "He loved me," Alex said. Then suddenly he felt a cold chill in the cheeks of his face. The fantasy died, and he knew that somewhere Sylvain was in his bed, and that in his dreams there was no Alex, no past. He was on that invisible ship; the ship that in sleep sails on either calm or rough seas, but which can, if the time comes, smash on unseen rocks, and then in oblivion, Sylvain would sink beneath the waves of all remembrance. So lost was Alex in his thoughts that he did not notice Paul had entered the room and was standing to one side by the open door, naked.

"I can't sleep," Paul said, making a slight move forward and then halting his advance.

"Do you want to sleep next to me?" Alex asked.

"Yes, but not for sex. I can assure you it's not for that."

"I believe you," Alex said, and made space for Paul to join him.

"I'm afraid," Paul said as he quickly slid between the sheets. Their bodies did not touch. "Let's go home." came the murmured request, and in answer, Alex reached out and brought Paul closer. He held his shaking body close to him, and they stayed like that in silence for a long while. Eventually, Alex felt the body beside him relax. Paul was asleep, and Alex stared at the alien objects in the room like a traveller who looks at his new surroundings with objective curiosity. Soon daylight would merge with the electric light of man and darkness would recede. Alex waited patiently for that to happen.

At breakfast, they behaved as if nothing had happened. Alex had gone out briefly to buy essentials, and they had a large meal. After they had finished, Alex asked, "Shall we go somewhere special today?"

Paul replied, "Show me a place I don't know."

"I will take you to one of my favourite quartiers—behind the Panthéon."

"The Panthéon?" Paul questioned.

"Yes, it's like a temple to the famous dead, but behind it, is the church of Saint-Étienne-du-Mont, which is truly beautiful, and from there, one side street leads to another where the poet Verlaine lived and died. It's like a village within the heart of Paris, and for many, it *is* the heart of Paris."

"Sounds cool. I'd like to see the heart of Paris," Paul replied.

"Well, it's not the heart of the city for all, just for some. The winding streets and the Place de la Contrescarpe, hold a special magic for those who can sense it, for those who want to return to it."

"And you do?"

"It depends upon how I feel. I would like to now."

"Then the heart of this city changes for you?"

"Yes," Alex replied, and he looked around the apartment as if it were already locked in the past. "My feelings shift."

They said nothing more until they were in the street. Neither of them wanted to take the Metro. The sun was shining. It was a brilliant day that had the illusion of summer without the heat—a typical tourists' day, and Alex could see that Paul appeared to be happy. Only once did Paul ask about Brighton and whether Alex would miss it. Alex closed the question by putting a finger over Paul's lips.

"Don't let's spoil it," he said.

In a backstreet on the left bank that Alex was sure he had never walked down in all the years he had lived in the city, they found a rather grubby shop which boasted of selling antiques but which looked more like a place for bric-a-brac. There were old paintings and torn posters in the window, and ancient dolls that were completely bald. It held the promise of the unexpected bargain. The bell rang as they entered, and a shy-looking woman came towards them.

"*Messieurs?*" she greeted them.

Alex stated that they were just browsing, and she nodded her head and retreated into a back room.

"She is very trusting," Paul whispered.

Before Alex could answer, he noticed a small pile of booklets, which on closer inspection turned out to be poetry from the 1950s. They were dusty and clearly had not been looked at in a long while.

"What a cemetery!" Alex said quietly and began to sort his way through them. He picked one out. The author was Greek. Alexis Palamas. He found three poems that he liked and read them twice. He then sat down on a nearby battered chair and called Paul over.

"I'd like you to hear these," he said. "They're from a small collection of poems. They're in French, but I'll read them to you in English. I can't say they are really good, but there is something in them making an attempt at the impossible."

Paul, who was holding a tin soldier, stared down at the booklet and said, "His name doesn't look French."

"No. Greek."

"But he writes in French?"

"I don't know. I've never heard of the writer before—so many are forgotten. Maybe he wrote in French, or maybe he was translated, but I imagine him to be a man who had seen a lot."

"I am listening," Paul said, and he looked genuinely interested.

"None of them have titles, and the words seem very naked on the page."

Paul glanced down. "It's only a couple of lines," he said.

Alex started reading.

> *Is the poem constant to its image?*
> *No, it is its own metamorphosis.*

"Is that all?" Paul asked.
"The second is longer."

The boy flannels his back standing on the shore
face averted from my gaze.
Is he thinking of the years to come
or is he immersed in the fleeting eternal moment?

Before Paul could comment, Alex turned to the third he had chosen.

Thoughts of elsewhere distract.
Better to be by the still stream
than to cross the unknown river.

"Yes," Paul said, smiling. "I like that one," and he wandered off, still holding the toy soldier tightly.

Alex read more of the poetry and then went in search of Paul who was looking at more toy soldiers.

"Reminds me of a set my dad used to have," Paul said. "He got rid of them in a jumble sale, and I was miserable for days."

"Didn't you tell him you wanted them?"

"No. I should have done. I was thirteen at the time. I'd given up on toys, and I was ashamed to tell him that the soldiers meant something to me."

"What did they mean to you?"

Paul was evasive and murmured, "Let's just say I liked them. Now, shall we go? Are you going to buy the poetry?"

"As long as I can buy these for you. What they mean to you is no business of mine. I don't want to probe, but they're in good condition, and it's a sunny day. Accept the gift."

Paul nodded his head, and the woman carefully wrapped each soldier and put them into a box.

As they walked up the Boulevard Saint-Michel, Paul paused and clutched at a nearby railing. He was having a giddy attack, and Alex guided him gently to a nearby café table. He then went to the counter and ordered a cognac for Paul.

"I hope it's not the fucking virus," Paul said as he sipped the drink.

Alex didn't reply. He looked around him. He knew that the fucking virus could be anywhere, and it was clear from the newspapers in the kiosks that the threat was growing daily. He feared too that the governments were holding back from putting actions into place, stalling on them, but he did not want to panic Paul with his thoughts.

"I was only joking," Paul said as he finished the cognac. "You know I have these attacks sometimes. Always have. Stress probably—when I am under too much strain. Anyway, I'm okay now. Let's go to this magic place you want to show me."

Slowly, and Alex made sure it was slow, they walked up to the Panthéon. Further on, the Place de la Contrescarpe was crowded, but the look on Paul's face showed that he liked it. Even in the cold sun, a group were playing jazz in the open space in the middle, and among all the cafés and restaurants that surrounded them, Alex noticed only one person wearing a mask.

"Can we sit down and listen?" Paul asked. "I'm not crazy about jazz, but it's somehow different here in the open air and under the sun. I always associate jazz with smoky clubs. I guess that's a cliché."

They sat on the terrace of the Contrescarpe Café, and Paul tapped his fingers on the table as he listened to the music. Alec leant back and realised he was weary. He had to talk seriously to Paul, but it could wait until the following day. The trees were bare, but the light, the sun, and the magic had attracted all the people around them. Will the same number be here next month and the month after, he wondered, but he smiled as Paul was smiling, and when the musicians paused he said, "I am glad you like it here," and as he said these words, he had a moment of clarity: Paul was quite simply a child who needed his toy soldiers for protection.

They stayed out for many hours. The sun set and the grey

shadows fell. Despite Paul's resistance, they took a taxi back to the apartment. In the taxi, Paul said, "We were all in danger there, weren't we? So close. It may be the last time—for a long time—that I will see so many people happy, but it was good to not feel panic for a while—panic for all of us, and fear."

The following day a drizzle fell upon the city. The kind of drizzle that depresses more than any other kind of weather. They ate their breakfast, and after they finished, it was Paul who spoke first.

"I want to leave today. Will you come with me or do I go alone?"

Alex, taken by surprise, was slow in replying. "What will you think of me if I stay?" he asked.

"That you are making a mistake. Can I speak the truth? What I believe is the truth."

"Of course."

"You are trying to escape old age and death by doing this. Run, run, run. Don't you know that death runs faster, or are you *still* the young man pretending that death is for others?"

"I believe in death alright," Alex said. "It's going to be all around us soon."

"Maybe, but in a village with strangers and nothing but strangers? At least in Brighton you would know me."

"I want my aloneness, Paul. I feel tense with others. Not just you. It's an accumulation of years and experiences that has brought me to this state. I want to be in a house that is my own, that I can walk freely in, in a place that is not going to pay much attention to me. Not that Brighton has for quite a while. I want the aloneness of it. Can you understand that?"

"Personally, I think you are throwing your life away."

"Let's not argue, Paul. I do have something to ask you. Call it a favour—just in case it all doesn't go as planned."

"What's that?"

"Take the keys I am going to give you. I would like you to stay in my flat until you have got on your feet. I will pay the landlord six months' rent. You won't have to worry about that. You can build up some savings for when you do move. We can talk often, and I will let you know how things are going."

"What if the transaction doesn't go through as you expect? There may be problems."

"If there are, I will tell you and I'll extend the rent money in Brighton if you need it."

Paul looked pale and sat on the floor. As if in denial, he turned on the television. The usual morning tripe that shows in every country blared out. Alex stared at it and felt numb.

"I have everything I need. I brought all my essential books with me. The rest can be sent over or got rid of eventually. In fact, take what you want, because unless things go really and truly wrong during this next six months, I will never return to Brighton."

"How can you be so *extreme*?" Paul cried out, a wail more than a cry, as if a blow had hit him. "Show me what you brought with you—your essential books, and what else?"

"There's nothing to show."

"Photos? Letters from the past? If they're not there, I certainly don't want to clear out your flat and stumble across them. I don't want to see them! I need to know that you have them with you. A man of your age must have them."

Alex turned off the television, and once again, silence filled the room. He looked at the wall where the drawing had been taken down and smashed. It was back in its place now, restored and none of the damage showed, but he thought again of Paul, of his mood swings and his harmful behaviour. He heard again the breaking glass and saw the look that Paul had had on his face. He then thought of his things in Brighton. What if Paul in a fit of anger or despair wreaked destruction there? Who would know? How much was he capable of destroying, and did it matter anyway? He knew in the ultimate analysis that none of that mattered.

"Show me the photos you are taking with you! I must know that you've got some feelings for your past. I know you haven't taken one of me. Up there behind the Panthéon, you could have. You could have wanted to remember, later in your life, that I had been, that I had existed. I didn't say anything, but I felt it, and I wanted to take one of you. I wanted a memory of you."

"Why?" Alex asked.

"Why? You ask why? It's because I care for you." Here he stopped and buried his head in his hands. He moved towards the window and stared out at the façades of the houses opposite. Alex went over and placed a hand on his shoulder.

"I don't want you to touch me anymore," Paul said.

"Do you care? Really?"

"Yes, I do. I don't call it love, but I've had better moments with you than anyone else I have had in my life. Now let's drop the subject, Alex."

Moved by this, Alex said, "Take a photo of me now."

"No. It's too late. But I will go back, and I will take care of your flat. I'm not sure I will live in it, but I'll visit it to check that no one has broken in and that everything's okay."

Alex sat on the sofa. He needed a drink—anything alcoholic as long as it took away the confusion that Paul was causing him, and had caused him since they had met. "Will you do something for me now?" he asked.

"What?" Paul turned around. His face was red. He stood in front of Alex, his hands hanging down to his sides. Alex noticed, perhaps for the first time, how beautifully formed they were. He saw the long, tapering fingers. He thought of a pianist's hands, and suddenly he wanted to reach out and touch them.

"What do you want me to do, Alex?"

"I want you to look in my suitcase—the one you didn't open. I want you to see what is there."

"In front of you?"

"Please. It's important."

Paul brought the suitcase from the bedroom and took out the books, one by one. There were about twenty, and then he noticed an envelope at the bottom of the case.

"What's that?" he asked.

"Have a look."

Paul tentatively took it out and found it was open.

"See what's inside," Alex murmured.

"But it's private—"

"All the more reason for you to see it."

Paul took out a photo. "I don't want to see it," and he put it face downwards, next to the case. He was kneeling on the floor, and Alex got off the sofa and knelt beside him. He knew that Paul would not touch it, so he turned over the photo himself.

"It's me," Paul said, staring down at his own image. "How did you? When did you?"

"One day, when you were not conscious of me."

Paul picked it up. The photo showed him sitting in the flat in Brighton. His head was tilted back against the chair he was sitting in. His face glowed, and he was smiling. His legs were stretched out, and the contours of his body clearly visible. It was a relaxed pose.

"Is this the only photo you took of me?" he asked, his voice trembling slightly.

"The only one."

"Then you—" and he stopped in mid-sentence.

"Yes, I do, Paul, but it's a confusion of sentiments. You see, I do not know what I truly feel about you. To call it love would be to use a word soiled by too much use, but I do feel. And at the last minute, before leaving the flat in Brighton and possibly leaving everything behind me, I was glad that I had put your photo in the suitcase. The rest of the photos of the past? Well, I destroyed most. Even the photos of—but I don't want to talk about that. I burned as much as I could of him in a night of fantasy and memory. But you—you, I wanted, to remind me that maybe there is no circle of barbed wire around me, no coldness of the heart or whatever cliché you want to call feeling. I will look at you often during the time that I remain in this apartment and once I arrive in Illiers-Combray. As I said, the house has been on the market a long time. Too long for them to reject my offer."

Paul said nothing, but carefully put the photo back in its envelope and placed it at the bottom of the suitcase.

"May I take one of you?" he asked, standing. He went over to his jacket and took out his mobile phone. "Stay where you are. I'd like to look at you and know that my photo is next to you." Alex smiled. "No, please don't smile. Nothing forced or false." Quickly he took the photo and put his mobile phone back in his jacket. "Give me the keys and take me to the station."

It was as if all Paris was in deep shadow as Alex took Paul to the Gare du Nord. They walked, and occasionally, Paul looked from side to side and asked questions as if gathering memories for the future. At the station, a ticket was bought, and as check-in was about to close, Paul asked Alex to walk away. He said he was not capable of saying goodbye. His face was drawn, and Alex, struck again by its beauty, wanted to caress it, but instead, smiled, turned quickly and walked away. He knew he would contact Paul once he was in Brighton, but beyond that who could know what the future held for either of them in the feverish time in which they lived.

****

Other published works by John Roman Baker

Novels
No Fixed Ground
The Dark Antagonist
The Paris Syndrome
The Sea and the City
The Vicious Age

The Nick & Greg Books
Nick & Greg
Time of Obsessions
Nick's House
Greg in Paris
Love & Cowardice
Greg at the Station

Short Stories
Brighton Darkness

Poetry
Cast Down
The Deserted Shore
Gethsemane
Poèmes à Tristan

Printed in Great Britain
by Amazon